Rethink, Redo, Rewired

Stay Strong
and
Keep Going.
Namaste,
Anthony A.

Rethink, Redo, Rewired

RETHINK, REDO, REWIRED: USING ALTERNATIVE TREATMENTS TO HEAL A BRAIN INJURY

ANTHONY AQUAN-ASSEE, M.Ed

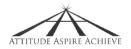

https://anthonyaquan-assee.com

National Library of Canada Cataloguing in Publication

Aquan-Assee, Anthony
Rethink, Redo, Rewired: Using Alternative Treatments to Heal a Brain Injury
Includes bibliographical references.
ISBN: 0973278234
ISBN 13: 9780973278231

Cover Design: Michael Aquan-Assee
Cover Art: Michael Aquan-Assee

iPhone is a registered trademark of Apple Inc.
Kangen Water® is a registered trademark of Enagic Co., Ltd.

Dedication

To my wife Jennifer.
It is with your strength that I could rewire.

Contents

Preface

THIS BOOK IS ABOUT MY discovery that I could help my brain and my body heal using some specific alternative treatments. I have learned to awaken my brain's healing capacity by using natural and noninvasive interventions. This empowered me to participate in my own healing and made the road to my recovery following a severe traumatic brain injury (TBI) a lot easier. The brain is not hardwired to remain the same, like a computer, but rather it continues to grow and change throughout one's life. These treatments that I used following three traumatic brain injuries may enable a person to pursue healing on their own rather than waiting for someone to do it for them. Health is much more than the absence of illness; it involves learning to live responsibly, which in essence is living in a way that promotes an internal state that helps to prevent illness.

The human body is a magnificent creation born with all the tools to heal itself. Being in charge of our health is what nature intended for us.

I acknowledge that doctors, surgeons, and other health-care professionals are important. In fact, I would not be alive if it were not for the skill of some great doctors and surgeons who helped save my life. However, a doctor's therapeutic bag of tricks often does not recognize that healing involves the mind, the body, and the spirit and is a process of becoming whole.

From an early age we are trained to go to the doctor when we believe something is wrong. This idea that doctors know best underestimates the extraordinary ability we have to heal ourselves. Wellness is trusting in the ability and desire of your mind and body to heal itself and make things better if it is given a chance.

Doctors are trained in disease, diagnosing, and treatment. We trust that modern medicine, with doctors as its soldiers, will win the war against disease, illness, and injury. Drugs are often the weapon of choice to help doctors win the war. The high-tech treatments available, as well as the innovations of drug companies, are intended to create new possibilities for patient care. Yet now, more than ever, many patients feel disconnected when it comes to their health care, like a helpless bystander.

The time has come for all the players in modern medicine to be more open to learning from their patients and not to discourage them from pursuing alternative treatments as an avenue toward healing. It is time for us to rethink, redo, and rewire ourselves to harness the mind, the body, and the spirit as allies in healing. We can heal ourselves.

This book is a guide and outlines what I have done to heal my brain and my body. I have researched, explored, and tried many alternative treatments and have written about those that have worked for me. The choice is now yours. My suggestion: try them out and see if they work for you. Always be sure to discuss with your doctor any treatments that you are thinking of using.

Please keep in mind that this book is about my own experiences. It is important to be aware that everyone's experiences will differ, as does the magnificent design and construction of people's brains.

This book has been written in the first person wherever possible. By telling my story, I hope to educate, motivate, and encourage others to explore the possibilities within to help heal themselves. My wife, mother, father, and other family members, as well as the professionals involved in my recovery, have all helped me write this book. Their contributions, words of encouragement, and never-ending support helped to lay the groundwork for me to Rethink, Redo, and Rewire.

In the words of St. Francis of Assisi,

"Start doing what's necessary; then do what's possible; and suddenly you are doing the impossible."

A Special Request from Anthony

Thank you for joining me in my book about using Alternative Treatments to Heal a Brain Injury.

I hope you benefit from reading my book.

If you enjoy my book, I would greatly appreciate a short review or testimonial and your permission to post this on my website. You can contact me on my website to send me your thoughts. Please visit https://anthonyaquan-assee.com. Your help in spreading the word is greatly appreciated. Reviews and testimonials from readers like you are so helpful to new potential readers searching for some help.

Thank you kindly,

Anthony Aquan-Assee

The Light

⤸

I LOOKED AROUND. I WAS surrounded by bright lights everywhere. I felt an extraordinary feeling of peace, comfort, and bliss.

Looking down, I saw myself swerving on my motorcycle to avoid the car. It was coming straight at me, and I couldn't avoid it. There was a head-on collision, and I wouldn't survive.

The car smashed into me, and suddenly here I was.

Where am I? Some kind of tunnel. Somewhere? Everywhere? Nowhere. It was all the same.

What's all this around me?

Never-ending streams of light were everywhere, and orbs of light were floating all around. I had never seen this before, but I wasn't scared. It was wonderful and very peaceful. Images of my life appeared right in front of me. I watched, remembered, and I understood. Everything that had happened in my life began to make sense.

Not just the accident, but also from the time when I was a child. It all was part of the plan for me for something bigger. Everything that had happened had prepared me for this day. It was all part of the same puzzle.

Now I get it, I thought. Then it all ended. I opened my eyes, and I was in the Neuro-Trauma Intensive Care Unit (ICU).

My girlfriend, Sherry, was standing at the bedside. She looked ecstatic and told me with great excitement that I was alive. I had been in a coma for two weeks, and I was a patient in the ICU at St. Michael's Hospital.

The doctors had told my family that there was little chance of my survival and that I wouldn't wake up from the coma. Even if I did, I would be a vegetable for the rest of my life and would need someone to take care of all my needs. There was no hope.

From that point on I had to understand what had happened to me.

What was it that I had just experienced? It was amazing and not of this world.

So began my unrelenting search to understand life as I had experienced it as a peaceful spirit.

This would take me to a place where I had to **Rethink**, **Redo**, and **Rewire** to understand my truth.

Introduction

⸻

My life changed completely after I sustained a severe traumatic brain injury in a horrific motorcycle accident.

In my rehabilitation I was told that I would never return to being a teacher again. I had sustained a severe brain injury, and my brain was too badly damaged.

Throughout my recovery, the doctors told me there was nothing they could do to help me cope with the problems associated with my brain injury. The challenge for me was to learn ways that would help me restore my body's ability to heal itself.

My recovery proceeded slowly, and then sixteen years later I sustained two more very serious traumatic brain injuries. That was the last straw. I had nowhere else to turn but to myself. The only solution the doctors had was to prescribe drugs.

Conventional medicine in North America is bound to the pharmaceutical industry. Doctors tend to rely on drug companies for information about the drugs they prescribe. They may not have adequate knowledge about possible alternatives to help treat their patients.

The side effects of the medications prescribed to me made my situation that much worse.

I refused to accept that there was no hope and so began my journey into the world of natural healing and alternative treatments.

In this book, I highlight several alternative treatments that have helped me to heal myself naturally. They enabled me to rely on my body's natural healing powers, as opposed to pharmaceutical drugs.

The Accident

It was September 23rd, 1997, and my life was going great. It was my second year of teaching in Toronto. I was a special education teacher for students who had severe learning disabilities and behaviour problems. It was a difficult class with frequent discipline issues. I loved the challenge of motivating my students never to give up so they could reach their potential. I was also the school's football coach, and my team had just qualified for the upcoming Toronto Football Championships.

That morning, I was jarred out of a deep sleep because an ambulance siren warned me to get out of the way.

I clutched the blankets, looked around, and felt a sudden moment of panic when I couldn't see my girlfriend.

Anxiously, I called out, "Sherry, where are you ? What's that noise?

"I'm downstairs," she replied. "Silly man, it's your alarm clock."

I cursed when I realized there wasn't a siren and then sat up in bed. My heart was still pounding. It was the same dream I'd been having for the past week, probably because my mother had recently told me about a motorcycle accident her friend's son had been in.

I cringed thinking about it, but even this wouldn't stop me from riding my motorcycle to school. It was brand new, and I wanted to show it to the other teachers.

Sherry startled me when she appeared at the door. "I'm making egg sandwiches, want one?"

"No," I said, pointing at the clock. "I can't be late for practice."

Sherry went back downstairs while I raced around the room, frantically gathering my stuff.

I showered, got dressed, and rushed down to the kitchen. An egg sandwich was waiting for me on the kitchen table.

"I don't have time to eat this," I grumbled. "I've got to get the team fully prepared for the championships. I can't be late."

Sherry charged over to the kitchen table and pulled out a chair. "Anthony, sit down and eat the egg sandwich that I've made for you, and don't waste it. You're always so impatient."

"There's no time to eat," I shouted, grabbing my backpack and storming out the front door.

The egg sandwich she made for me would remain on the counter uneaten. This was a decision that would change the course of my life forever.

"The roads we take are more important than the goals we announce. Decisions determine destiny."

—Frederick Speakman

STARTING POINT & THE TRAIN STATION

I flooded the engine, trying to start my motorcycle. I cursed, worried that I'd be late for the practice.

It took me several minutes to get the engine started. In hindsight, perhaps I should have given up, but it's not in my nature to do that.

The traffic on the main road moved steadily. It didn't take long before I approached the major intersection in front of the train station. I entered the intersection, and suddenly a car raced through the intersection and smashed into me. My motorcycle was destroyed, and I was sent soaring through the air into the next phase of my life.

Looking down, I saw myself swerving on my motorcycle to avoid the car. The accident happened, and suddenly I was a spirit in the sky looking down a tunnel filled with a very bright light.

Even though I was witnessing an accident that was going to change the course of my life, I felt very calm, as if I were merely an observer. The accident would give me the opportunity to rethink, redo, and rewire myself. I would learn from my mistakes and work to rectify them. But it would require a tremendous effort for me to start over again. In order to continue to go forward, I could never give up.

"Never, never, never, never give up."

—Winston Churchill

The Accident Scene

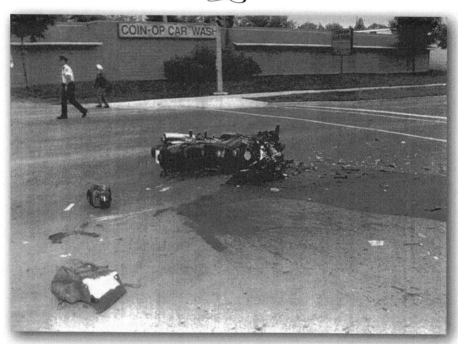

Anthony's destroyed motorcycle at the scene of the accident.

THE ACCIDENT SCENE

The paramedics arrived at the scene to find me crumpled on the street some distance from my motorcycle. My helmet was still on my head, and I was bleeding from my eyes, my ears, my nose, and my mouth. All signs of a very serious brain injury.

After careful examination, the paramedics discovered that I wasn't breathing, and I didn't have a pulse. They called for an air ambulance and then went to work trying to revive me. There didn't appear to be much hope for my survival. My brain had been deprived of oxygen for some time. In addition to my severe head injury, I also appeared to have sustained many serious internal injuries. The paramedics continued to work frantically on me as I was transported to the closest hospital. But this hospital wasn't equipped to deal with the extent of my injuries, so I was then taken by air to the trauma unit at St. Michael's Hospital in Toronto.

THE PHONE CALL

That morning, my mother, Josephine Aquan-Assee received the phone call every mother dreads. She was a grade two teacher and was called out of her class to take a phone call.

Josephine rushed into the office, worried and concerned.

"Who is calling me?" Teaching a grade two class was extremely busy work, and a phone call was a disruption.

"I don't know. They didn't say," said the secretary, quietly handing the phone to her.

"Hello," Josephine said.

"Ma'am, this is Officer Wilson with Peel Regional Police."

Josephine gulped, and her heart sank.

"I'm sorry to inform you but your son, Anthony, has been involved in a very serious motorcycle accident."

Josephine's thoughts immediately flashed to the scene of an accident she had noticed out of the corner of her eye while driving to school that morning. Her school was close to where my girlfriend lived, but she hadn't known who was involved in the accident.

The traffic had been redirected, and it appeared to be a serious accident. She recalled saying some silent prayers as she drove by. Now this.

Without another word from the officer, she knew the accident she had driven by that morning had involved me.

With a feeling of dread Josephine quietly asked, "Is he going to be okay?"

"I don't know," said the officer, "you had better get to St. Michael's Hospital ASAP."

Josephine hung up the phone in a state of shock. She then called her husband, Kenneth.

St. Michael's Hospital

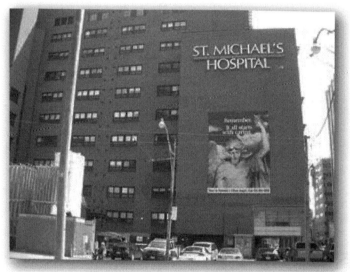

St. Michael's Hospital, Toronto

Josephine and Kenneth were both quiet during the drive to the hospital, thinking about all the "what ifs" of the situation. They wondered what was happening to their son and where he was in the hospital.

Josephine had a feeling of dread. She prayed that I was safe and in good hands. Kenneth gripped the steering wheel, concentrating hard on the drive. He drove quietly, his mind racing with a million thoughts.

When they got to St. Michael's, Josephine saw an ambulance at the emergency entrance, and her heart sank even lower. When they got to the parking lot, all the closest spots were reserved, and they had to park quite a distance away. As soon as they got out of the car, Josephine mumbled something and then started to run. Kenneth ran after her. When they ran by the ambulance, Josephine stumbled and reached out, grabbing Kenneth's hand. Gasping, panting, and crying, they held each other as they stumbled up the steps through the emergency doors.

There were many people standing inside the emergency room as Josephine and Kenneth approached the reception desk.

"Anthony Aquan-Assee?" said Josephine to the female attendant sitting behind the desk.

The attendant didn't respond immediately, and then after what seemed like an eternity, she looked up.

"Who are you?"

"Anthony's parents," whispered Josephine. Her anxiety was almost unbearable, and she struggled to control her quavering voice. "I was told that my son was in an accident and was brought here. Is he alright?"

The fear of the unknown tightened her throat, brought a throbbing pain to her head, and caused her eyes to well up with tears.

The attendant, apparently oblivious to this turmoil, said, "Please go sit in the waiting room. Someone will come to speak to you about your son as more information becomes available."

Afraid to ask, Josephine whispered, "Is he dead?"

Seeing the fear in her eyes, the attendant replied quietly, "No, but you will have to go and wait for more information."

"Until the day of his death, no man can be sure of his courage."

-—Jean Anouilh, 1920–1987

7

THE WAIT

Discouraged, Kenneth and Josephine went with the nurse around the corner to the waiting room. Josephine anxiously scanned the gurneys in the hallway to see if I was lying on one of them. She didn't see me or see or hear any clues that indicated I was nearby. Josephine desperately wanted to help me but knew my fate was in the hands of the doctors at St. Michael's.

The waiting room was very untidy, with coffee cups and water bottles lying everywhere, but the room and the voices of the other people ceased to exist as Josephine and Kenneth struggled with the need to know what was happening to their son.

Several hours passed before a doctor came to speak to them.

His eyes had dark circles under them, and his arms were clutched tight across his chest. "Are you Mr. and Mrs. Aquan-Assee?"

"Yes," they blurted out. They had been slumped against each other.

"Anthony is in surgery right now. He's in very serious condition. You will have to wait to find out anything more."

Josephine gasped, and Kenneth croaked, "What?"

Tears ran from their eyes.

"Is he going to be okay?" whispered Josephine.

"I'm sorry," the doctor said, "I can't tell you what will happen, but I will be sure to keep you up to date as soon as more information becomes available."

The doctor walked away scribbling on his clipboard, his head bowed sadly.

I was in neurosurgery to stop the bleeding in my brain. The CAT scan had revealed very serious brain damage.

The truth was that the doctor wasn't ready to tell my parents that in his twenty years as a critical care physician, he had never seen someone survive such a horrific accident.

Following this initial surgery, I remained in the operating room for additional surgery. The surgeons had to remove my ruptured spleen and repair my lacerated intestines and liver. They also had to repair my ruptured femoral artery, the main artery of my leg. The surgeons worked quickly and performed a blood transfusion to stop me from bleeding to death.

Josephine and Kenneth sat in the waiting room in a state of shock, fearing the worst.

Josephine was in a daze. It had been a very long wait with little information. She guessed that I was in serious condition.

After an endless eight-hour wait, a doctor came out and told them I was being taken to the ninth floor Neuro-Trauma Intensive Care Unit (ICU). They would be re-evaluating my condition shortly.

Kenneth and Josephine went up to the ninth floor, feeling like robots, numb, devoid of emotion. As they exited the elevator, they saw a room filled with people, as well as people sitting in the blue chairs that lined the hallway. There was no room for privacy. In the waiting room, a young couple sat beside an older woman. Their faces were sombre, and the silence was interrupted by the fitful coughing of a man sitting in the hallway.

On the wall outside the waiting room was a sign that read, "*Please use buzzer to contact the ICU.*"

Josephine gestured to Kenneth and then, determined to see her son, extended her finger toward the buzzer. She stopped when she heard a cheerful voice behind her.

"Hello, can I help you find someone?"

A man wearing a green jacket sat at a desk. The sign on the desk read, "*Volunteer on Duty.*"

"We're trying to find our son, Anthony. A doctor told us downstairs that he was being brought to the Neuro-Trauma Intensive Care Unit. Are we in the right place?" asked Josephine.

The young man pulled out a sheet of paper with names on it and examined it carefully. "What's his last name?" he asked.

"Aquan-Assee," Josephine replied.

"Ah, yes, here he is. He's in bed number 10. First, let me check with the nurse to see if it's okay for you to go inside and see him."

He left Josephine and Kenneth standing there, exasperated that they had to wait again before they could see me. After several minutes of restless waiting while the hallway filled with people and then emptied again, the volunteer finally returned.

Horror in the ICU

Josephine and Kenneth gasped in horror. They stood beside the bed, eyes wide and open-mouthed when they saw me. Josephine reached out and grabbed Kenneth's arm to steady herself. There were no words to describe what they saw. I was the size of the bed. My body was swollen, battered, and bloody. I looked like a giant blow-up doll. My head was shaved and larger than a basketball. Thick surgical staples held together a massive incision that ran down the side of my head, looking almost as if it were a train track.

The train track-like incision continued down the middle of my abdomen. Just above on my chest were many pads that connected to a computer monitor with several waves oscillating on it.

Josephine cringed and turned away. I was unrecognizable. My face was black and blue and so swollen and deformed.

The bones in my face had been crushed. Kenneth breathed a deep sigh and reached out to hold his wife as tears ran down their faces.

The nurse at the bedside introduced herself. She explained what they had done with me in surgery and why I looked so swollen.

Kenneth asked the nurse what all the equipment that surrounded my bed was used for.

She nodded and pointed at the tube in my mouth. "We've got him intubated now."

"What's intubated?" Kenneth asked.

"It means that we've inserted a tube into his trachea — his windpipe — and the ventilator is breathing for him."

Josephine gasped, "He can't breathe?"

The nurse gently shook her head. "No, not right now." She reached out and lightly touched Josephine's hand. "He's in a deep coma, and the life support machine is keeping him alive."

Josephine and Kenneth stood by the bed, sobbing and holding each other in complete shock.

Nothing could have prepared them for this. With the fear of death in her eyes, my mother reached out to hold my hand, hoping I would open my eyes and look at her. Seeing the look of desperation on Josephine's face, the nurse quietly whispered to her, "Anthony won't be able to respond to you right now."

Kenneth and Josephine left the ICU and went into the hallway to regain their composure. How could anyone survive what their son had gone through?

A grey-haired doctor finally appeared and approached them slowly, his white coat tightly buttoned up as if to guard against the sadness so prevalent in the ICU. He introduced himself to my parents as the Trauma Team Leader on duty in the ICU.

"Your son has been in a horrific accident and is in extremely serious condition. I would suggest that you prepare for the worst." After a pause he gently suggested, "We don't know if he'll live through the night, but you should go home and get some rest. You'll need all your strength in the next few days."

When Josephine and Kenneth returned the next day, nothing had changed. I was still in a very deep coma.

Each day was a journey down a road never travelled. At first my family felt fear, anxiety, depression, and despair, but they never gave up hope; they always believed there was some. They sat by my bedside every day and night hoping to see some sign that I was still inside the lifeless mass of battered flesh lying on the bed. They worked co-operatively, focusing totally on me. The day-to-day routine of their lives was set aside so they could be there for me. They hoped and prayed and then prayed some more.

The days turned into weeks, and their feelings of desperation intensified.

Josephine and Kenneth knew they needed to have a plan in place so that when I came out of the coma I would receive the maximum support. Pictures of Sherry, Jonathan, and Michael (My two younger brothers), Jasmin (My older sister), as well as Josephine and Kenneth, were placed on the IV stand beside my bed. They wanted me to see them when I opened my eyes and to know they were with me in this foreign environment.

After two weeks, there still wasn't any sign of life.

The Decision

I had been in a coma for over two weeks when the doctors on the trauma team asked my mother to meet them for a case conference in the private "quiet room" just outside the ICU.

Fear and uncertainty followed her as she dragged herself to the quiet room. She took a deep breath and knocked. The door opened slowly. The entire table was surrounded by doctors she had seen in the ICU.

"Good morning, Josephine," said the grey-haired doctor, closing the door behind her and pulling out a chair for her. "We wanted you present at the case conference to discuss Anthony's progress."

Josephine just stared and didn't say a word.

"Anthony remains in a vegetative state and has been unresponsive to any sensory stimulation for over two weeks now." He pointed at the CAT scan on the wall.

"As we can see from this scan, it is unlikely your son will ever emerge from the coma, and even if he does, he will probably be a vegetable for the rest of his life."

His words echoed in her mind. *Vegetable, vegetable, vegetable...*

He turned to the other doctors, who were nodding in agreement.

Josephine swallowed hard then shook her head. "No," she barked. "No." She knew what they were getting at. "I know my son, and I know that he's still alive," she said, pointing to her heart.

"Yes, but remember," the doctor said gently, "Anthony is being kept alive by the life support machine."

The doctors stood up to let her grieve in private. Just before he closed the door, the grey-haired doctor turned around.

"Don't expect too much, and take some time to think about the quality of life Anthony would have wanted."

The doctor left, and just like her son, Josephine was all alone.

The next day, Josephine and Kenneth walked into the ICU determined to prove to themselves and the doctors that I was still alive and "in there."

The doctors stood at the bedside doing their assessments. They stepped aside so Kenneth could approach me.

"Anthony!" he shouted. "Are you in there, Anthony? Move your feet! Move your toes!" Josephine and the doctors watched and said nothing. Nothing happened. Just the sound of the life support machine breathing for me. It was more like a wheezing sound and not human breathing. Machine breathing. They waited some more, and then suddenly to everyone's amazement, my toe moved. Then I gripped my father's hand and squeezed it. My father gasped and turned to see the doctors' reaction. "He squeezed my hand!" he shouted.

Then my arm moved. The grey-haired doctor told me to open my eyes. My eyeballs were moving beneath my closed eyelids, clearly struggling to open. The doctor completed a few more assessments that all showed I was beginning to emerge from the coma.

With his face flushed and his hands in his pockets, the doctor turned to Josephine and Kenneth.

"It looks like we were premature in our diagnosis." He turned hastily and quickly walked off. Josephine and Kenneth were ecstatic. I was alive.

Debt of Gratitude

All the assessments and observations the doctors had available to them indicated there was no hope. The computer equipment also showed that I was unresponsive and there was little chance of me regaining consciousness. What nobody realized is that nothing is impossible. There are some things in life that don't have a "scientific" explanation. Through the doctors' expertise, their devotion to saving lives, and the fantastic care I received in the ICU, the impossible became possible.

Fear and Confusion

I opened my eyes and woke up from what seemed like an eternity. I was later told that I had been in a deep coma for two weeks. Where was I? What was I doing here? Why were all these tubes in my body? The physical pain was overwhelming and the fear was paralyzing. What had happened to me? Sherry was standing beside my bed, and her face lit up when I opened my eyes. Her eyes jumped for joy as she told me that I was alive. She gently told me that I had been in a motorcycle accident and was in St. Michael's Hospital. The questions racing through my mind were endless. I kept slipping in and out of consciousness, unable to concentrate on something for longer than a few seconds. It felt as though my brain had a short circuit, turning on and off every few seconds. I knew my brain wasn't working properly, and it scared me. Knowing I couldn't communicate, Sherry moved closer to me, hoping her presence would give me some security.

The pain that throbbed through my body was excruciating and was aggravated by the many tubes coming out of my throat, chest, and abdomen. They were all draining fluids that were coming out of me. It felt like an elephant was sitting on my chest, splitting it apart. I wanted someone to help me, but I was unable to speak. It felt like I was trapped in hell.

Sherry couldn't contain her excitement and ran out of the ICU to find Josephine and Kenneth. The day they had all been praying for had finally come. Josephine and Kenneth were talking to the social worker when Sherry ran up.

"Jo, Ken, come quickly," she shouted. "Anthony just opened his eyes. Come and see!"

Josephine's mouth dropped open. "Really!"

They all ran to the ICU, hoping my eyes would still be open. When they got to my bedside, my eyes were still open.

"Hi, Anthony," Josephine whispered. "We're all here."

My eyes remained open for only a few minutes, after which I lapsed back into a coma again.

Anxious and frustrated, Josephine and Kenneth eventually decided to go home and rest, hoping there would be a change the next day.

The next day, they walked into the ICU hopeful that I was awake.

Josephine sighed and gripped Kenneth's hand when she saw me.

My eyes were closed.

The nurse came over and gently placed her hand on Josephine's shoulder.

"He's remained unconscious and hasn't moved at all."

Just then the heart surgeon appeared. "Hi," he said, nodding to Josephine and Kenneth. "I came by to assess Anthony. We have to make sure he is well enough to proceed with the heart surgery tomorrow."

I had broken my ribs in the accident from the impact of the car hitting me. The broken bones cut through my heart, as well as my lungs, leaving them badly damaged.

Ever since I had arrived in the ICU, there had been a battle between the neurosurgeons and the heart surgeons. The neurosurgeons were trying to save my badly damaged brain, while the heart surgeons were trying to save my badly damaged heart.

But the neurosurgeons didn't want to take the chance of any additional surgery, as it would most likely kill me. My brain was swelling out of control, and if I were put under anaesthetic and connected to the heart-lung machine, they believed I would die.

The neurosurgeons had to wait and see. If they were going to declare me brain-dead, then any surgery before this would have been pointless.

But now things were different. I had opened my eyes and showed that I was still in there. Just as Josephine had stated.

The heart surgeon stood up and turned to Josephine. "Anthony's breathing is laboured," he said as he removed his stethoscope. There might be something wrong. I'll have to re-assess him tomorrow."

Josephine sat down and put her head in her hands. Tears rolled down her face.

The next day, my eyes opened, but they didn't remain open for very long. When they were open I would only stare vacantly straight ahead. Nothing registered, and I didn't respond to anything, only empty staring with no recognition. Later that morning the heart surgeon came by to check up on me again. There was definitely a problem with my breathing. The surgery had to be postponed, since it was too dangerous right then.

Jonathan and Michael came the next day to visit me. Just as they all sat down, my leg kicked out at the nurse as she stood at the bedside.

It was as if I was telling her to leave. My wild behaviour then intensified as my family helplessly looked on in horror. I had now reached up and pulled out my breathing tube. Next, the heart monitor connections were ripped off. My behaviour was like that of a wild caged animal. My family was quickly ushered out of the ICU so the nurses and doctors could attend to me.

The following day, my eyes remained closed and there were no signs I was in there. The effort I'd expended from the chaotic events of the previous day must have drained all my energy. It appeared that I had lapsed back into a coma. No signs even when the nurse applied a painful stimulus to see if I would move or open my eyes. Nothing, no movement, no sound, nothing registered, not even on the EEG machine, which registered my brain waves.

For the next several days I would slip in and out of consciousness. I was unable to keep my eyes open and focus my attention on anything for longer than a few seconds. It quickly became apparent that my recovery was going to be a long ordeal.

My mother and father continued to receive many phone calls from my friends, who were all anxious to see me. Sam, Mark, Chris, Rami, Neil, and many others all wanted to come by. But right now it was a priority to reduce the amount of stimulation on my brain so that I could rest and heal.

My mother told my friends that I needed to rest and that she would call them when I was ready for visitors.

THE MAN WHO BROUGHT PARDON TO INJURY

Sam looked sadly down at the tickets in his hand. He missed me and had hoped he would be able to see me soon. Sam and I had bought the tickets two months ago as soon as we found out that Dr. Wayne Dyer was coming to speak in Toronto.

Dr. Dyer was a psychologist and a motivational speaker that we both greatly respected and admired. He had written many books that we really enjoyed; it was very important to both of us to follow his words of wisdom and motivation.

Anthony will be so sad that he missed this, Sam thought. *I'll go and hopefully be able to speak to Dr. Dyer.*

After the presentation, Sam lined up with hundreds of other fans, hoping to speak to the man known as "The Father of Motivation." The line progressed slowly, until finally there was only one other person in front of Sam. He stood anxiously waiting, hoping he could find a way to help his friend.

When it was his turn, Dr. Dyer shook Sam's hand vigorously.

"Hello, Dr. Dyer." Sam smiled. "My name is Sam, and I'm a big fan of yours. My friend Anthony is also a big fan, but he couldn't come here today. He was in a bad motorcycle accident and now he is in a coma at St. Michael's Hospital. It's only just a few blocks from here." He stopped to pause and collect his thoughts.

What is the best way to ask him? Sam thought.

"I was wondering," Sam continued, "would you be able to go there and visit him? I know he would love it. He's read so many of your books and was planning on coming here today."

Dr. Dyer's first thought was about the plane he had to catch later that day. He often received requests to help people, but he didn't think he would have time to go to the hospital.

Thinking of the wonderful things he had heard about Dr. Dyer, Sam tried again with a little more urgency. "Would you please just be in his presence? Just bring your energy."

Dr. Dyer thought for a moment. Sam's plea reminded him that life gives to life.

"Yes," he said. "I'll go." Dr. Dyer left the auditorium early so he could stop at the hospital on his way to the airport. He took the elevator to the ICU where Anthony lay.

A nurse greeted him as he walked in.

"Hello, can I help you?"

"Ah, yes, I'm here to see Anthony," said Dr. Dyer.

"Are you a doctor?" asked the nurse.

"Yes," he replied, even though he might not have been the kind of doctor who generally worked in the ICU. She pointed to my bed, and he walked over. Dr. Dyer could see how badly damaged my body was. Would I live much longer? Dr. Dyer began to pray and meditate at the bedside, surrounding my body with a healing energy. The healing energy was meant to bring pardon to my injured body.

As he left the hospital for the airport, Dr. Dyer thought that if I could connect to the healing energy, one day I would be able to walk out of the hospital.

From that point on, Dr. Dyer included me in his daily prayers.

Josephine and Kenneth arrived at the hospital a short time later and were overjoyed to hear that Dr. Dyer had visited me. They had always encouraged me to follow his work, and now he had gifted me with his presence.

The next day, my eyes were open when my mother arrived at the hospital.

Her heart went to her throat and she gasped when she saw me.

"Hi, Anthony," she whispered. It had been four weeks since I arrived in the ICU, and this was the first time I actually looked at her. My eyes remained open, and it looked like I was listening. My mother spoke slowly and clearly and told me where I was and what happened. My eyes stayed open for several minutes, but again they closed and I was unconscious again. At least my eyes had stayed open for longer.

OPEN-HEART SURGERY

The next day, I was wheeled to the operating room.

My family, friends, and some of my coworkers huddled together in the waiting room. I was strong enough for the open-heart surgery, but it was still very risky.

Eight hours later, the surgeon came out of the operating room to speak with my parents.

"If I had known just how badly damaged his heart was, I wouldn't have waited so long to do this," said the surgeon.

"Why," questioned Josephine. "What was wrong?"

"His aorta was hanging on by only a thread of skin," said the surgeon. "It could have gone anytime, and that would have been it. We also couldn't repair his heart valves," he added.

Josephine gulped and grabbed Kenneth's arm. "What does this mean?"

The surgeon reached out and touched her hand. "He's okay right now. I held your son's heart in my hands. I would never let anything happen to him. But he's going to need a valve replacement when he is older."

Josephine and Kenneth went with the surgeon to the recovery room.

Two weeks later I was taken to the operating room for lung surgery. There had never been a lung surgery at St. Michael's Hospital, so a thoracic surgeon was brought in from another nearby hospital to complete this surgery.

My lungs were badly damaged, and the surgeon initially thought that my left lung would have to be removed. Thankfully, they were able to save it.

During the next month I underwent several other major operations, the first of which was plastic surgery to repair the broken bones in my face. I had broken my nose, my jaw, and my cheekbone, as well as the bone above my left eye. This surgery was a very delicate procedure necessary to prevent loss of sight in my left eye. The bones in my face were held together by metal plates, screws, and wires. I had also broken my right knee and torn all the ligaments in my knee. This required knee surgery, and after that there was throat surgery. After these major surgeries, the subtle, early signs of internal bleeding were missed resulting in the need for emergency surgery. My femoral artery had ruptured once again.

All the doctors said it was a miracle that I survived this accident. After being a patient in the ICU for two months, another miracle took place: I was transferred to the main floor of the neurosurgical ward. I spent the next month as a patient there.

NEUROSURGICAL WARD

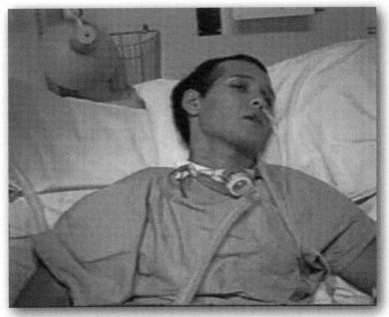

In my room on the neurosurgical ward

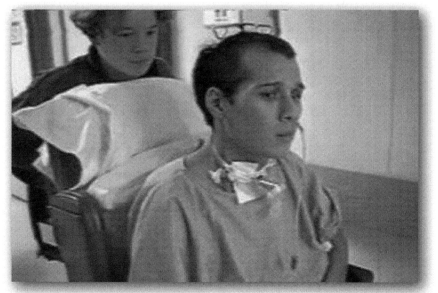

My brother Mike pushing my wheel chair on the neurosurgical ward

Following this, I was transferred to a rehabilitation hospital for neuro-rehabilitation. It was there where I began the journey to Rethink, Redo, and Rewire to help heal my brain.

"The things which hurt, instruct."

—Benjamin Franklin

Another Accident

IT WAS WEDNESDAY, AND I had woken up with a start. The alarm had gone off, and I wasn't even ready yet. This never happened, since I was always up before the alarm. Rarely did I sleep more than four hours, even with all the sleep medication I was taking. The doctors said it was because of my brain injury. They told me that sleep problems were very common after such an injury.

It had been sixteen years since my accident, but it felt like it was only yesterday. My memory was horrible, as were my attention and concentration. Everything was a huge challenge for my brain, and I worked tirelessly to keep my disability invisible.

I was exhausted, but I couldn't be late! I was never late for anything. Grabbing my clothes and sprinting downstairs, I got ready to start my run. It had rained during the night, and there were puddles all over the road, making it wet and slippery. By this time water was seeping into the cracks of my shoes, and my socks were soaked. It didn't matter, since I had a time to beat.

I shook my feet to get rid of the leaves clinging to my wet shoes. Ever since I was a kid I had never lost a race, and today the race was against my stopwatch. I wanted to beat my best time to prove to myself that I could do whatever I wanted.

Just like clockwork, I rounded the first corner by 6:00 a.m. The cold November morning air helped me to feel a bit more awake, and all that could be heard was the sound of my shoes slapping the pavement. It seemed like me and the chirping birds were the only ones awake. If I could face this challenge I had set for myself, I would feel more confident to deal with the challenge I was facing at my school. My Teacher's Performance Appraisal (TPA) was coming up soon, and I would have to demonstrate competence in my classroom with my principal watching me as I taught a lesson. This worried me a lot, since I had a unusually difficult class and my brain injury made it very challenging for me to keep track and remember all the things going on, especially when I was always so tired.

More than anything else, I wanted to accept and believe in myself without the constant reminder of being a brain injury survivor. If I could set a new personal best in my running, that would be the proof I needed to believe I could achieve anything I wanted. All other achievements had been forgotten.

The sound of my feet hitting the pavement became louder as I rounded the final corner. I blistered down the street to my house, even though my knee was killing me and my lungs were burning and gasping for air. I bent over on the driveway, struggling to catch my breath. A surge of exhilaration rushed through me as I looked at my watch. I had just set a new personal best.

TPA

Lunchtime was coming soon when the principal poked her head into my classroom. Her eyes lingered for a moment on my students fooling around, then she turned her attention to me.

"Are you going to be around during lunch?" she asked.

"No," I said.

She frowned. "I wanted to discuss your teacher's performance appraisal."

I nodded. "I'm going out at lunch. Can we do it when I return?"

"Okay," she said. "Don't forget, your TPA is in two weeks."

She turned and left. The reminder made my stomach turn.

I swallowed and turned my attention back to my students.

The students were a strange mix. Some were givers and the rest were takers. The givers liked to help out in class, while the takers contributed very little. Instead, they tried to get as much as they could from everyone else, and rarely did they follow any rules.

The givers were fidgeting with their lunch bags in their chairs. The takers were all standing, fooling around by the class aquarium.

"Back to your seats! Get away from the aquarium!" I ordered.

Only the students sitting in their chairs looked at me. The rest of the students continued to fool around by the aquarium. They refused to listen.

I was tired of spending so much time on behaviour management.

Just then two boys who had been standing across from each other began to call each other names.

Standing together, they looked like the exact opposites. David's long hair ran halfway down his back, and his imposing frame dwarfed tiny Quade, who had short, curly hair. They didn't like each other and often got into fights.

Harsh words quickly turned into a commotion. David's height made him look even more imposing. Soon the pandemonium spilled out into the hallway, with their friends following and taking sides.

I stood there in shock and needed some help.

"Alex," I shouted, pointing at the wall, "press the office intercom button."

He quickly jumped up and jabbed the button.

"Yes, Mr. A," said the office secretary, oblivious to the outburst in the hallway.

"Please get the principal to deal with the fight going on outside my classroom."

I turned and walked over to the class reading area.

"Come join me." I motioned to the remaining five students. They were sitting huddled at their desks and looked relieved when I called them over. My main concern was to make sure they were safe.

Just then the principal's piercing voice could be heard over the shouting in the hallway. Everything went quiet.

Thank goodness, I thought. Just in time for the lunch bell.

After dismissing my students, I flopped down in my comfy teacher's chair. I sighed and then took a deep breath.

A few minutes later, I ran out to my car to go to a store during the lunch hour. Hopefully this would give me enough time to refresh my brain and return to school ready for round number two.

Once back at school, I walked toward the chain-link fence that surrounded the school. The afternoon sun glinted on the tall metal gate that stood in front of the school doors.

The gate was heavy, so I forcefully pushed on it. The gate quickly swung forward for a bit, but then even more quickly, it swung right back and smashed me on the head. It felt as if someone had just bashed my head with a metal baseball bat. I was knocked unconscious and fell face-first to the ground. When I awoke, the pain in my head was severe and blood was dripping down my face. I slowly crawled to the school's front door and was helped inside. The principal and the other teachers were horrified when they saw me. My wife, Jen, was called and arrangements were made for me to go to the hospital.

Once at the hospital I was immediately taken for a CAT scan of my head. My head was hurting so much that I was unable to answer any questions. The light was blinding and made my headache worse, so I kept my eyes closed and then fell asleep.

When I awakened, Jen was sitting beside me, resting her head against my arm.

"I'm awake," I said to her.

Jen looked up, and with fear in her eyes she asked, "Do you know where you are?"

"Hospital." It was difficult to think, and I closed my eyes again and drifted off.

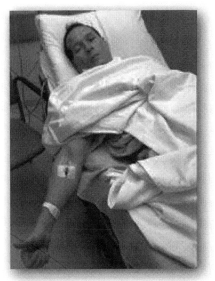

Anthony in the Emergency (2013)

When I opened my eyes, a man in a white coat was staring at me. A pen and a small notebook poked out of his white coat pocket.

"Hello, Anthony," said the man. "I'm going to do a quick check-up on you." He then shone a light in my eyes.

I winced at the brightness and blinked until the bright spots in my eyes went away.

"Okay, now please touch your nose with your finger."

"Good," he said when I had done that.

"Now please touch my left finger with your right finger."

I struggled.

Which one is my right finger?

I was worried he would think I was stupid.

He repeated this with my left finger touching his right finger. Again I was lost.

Which one is his right finger?

The man smiled and then said, "I'm Dr. Niaga. I'm the emergency doctor." He looked down at some papers and then said, "You've got some lacerations on your forehead. Probably from the metal gate hitting your head."

I watched him talk and had to concentrate extremely hard to understand what he was saying.

"The lump on your head is probably from when your head hit the ground. Ice your head and the swelling will go down, but you'll likely see some bruising soon."

He pointed at my head. "The good news is that the CAT scan doesn't show any bleeding in your brain. But because you sustained a concussion, you will need observation."

Jen gasped. "Is a concussion the same as a brain injury?" she asked.

"Yes," said the doctor, nodding. "A concussion is a traumatic brain injury, just not the same as a severe one."

He pulled a pen from his white coat pocket and started writing something on the papers he was holding. "It's too early to say how this will affect Anthony's brain. He's going to need a lot of rest now."

Jen sighed then reached out and grabbed my hand. "Anthony already sustained a severe traumatic brain injury in a motorcycle accident back in 1997. Will this affect him?"

The doctor smiled reassuringly at Jen. "Anthony must have a strong brain. However, the effects of multiple concussions over time can result in long-term problems. Only time will tell how this will affect Anthony."

He folded the papers he had been writing on and handed them to Jen. "These are the papers Anthony must take to his employer, since he was injured at work."

He turned to face me. "I want you to get lots of rest and take as much time off from work as you need. Recovery from a concussion can take days, or it can take weeks. Don't return to work until you are symptom-free."

The doctor turned back to Jen. "It's very important that you monitor him closely in the next few days. Anthony's brain will heal in the next few weeks, and make sure he gets a lot of rest."

He continued to speak to Jen, but I was unable to focus on what he was saying. I stopped listening. I just wanted to go home.

When we arrived home, more snow began falling.

I was too groggy to help Jen shovel the driveway and instead fell asleep on the couch.

Day 1

The next day I woke up at 5:00 a.m. after having slept for only three hours. I had great difficulty falling asleep and was up until two in the morning. I was so tired when I woke up, and my head was pounding.

When Jen was getting ready to leave for work, she came to me with a worried look. "Anthony, I don't think you should be out of bed."

"I'm exhausted but I can't sleep," I whispered.

"Well, just lie down in bed, and maybe you'll fall asleep. You shouldn't be walking on the stairs in your groggy state. Imagine what would happen if you fell and hit your head again."

She led me to bed and tucked me in. "Here," she said as she passed me the phone. I'll call you from work to make sure you're okay."

I nodded.

My brain felt like it was stuck in a fog. How was I going to call my work to take a sick day?

Lucky for me, Jen and I could read each other's faces and body language like we were reading a book. Words were not needed.

I handed Jen the phone and pointed to my head.

She made the call to my work and told them that I would not be coming in for the rest of the week.

Jen placed the phone back down on my bedside table then leaned down to kiss me. "I'll call you every couple hours. Keep this phone beside you at all times."

Then she left, and I was alone with my thoughts.

I couldn't believe it. Another brain injury. This was my third chance at life and my first day in my new life.

I looked at my watch, 7:00 a.m., Thursday. Time ceased to matter to me. The only thing that mattered to me was that this was the first day after my second brain injury: Day 1.

Now if only I could get some more sleep.

Day 2

It had been two days since my accident, and it didn't look like there was any relief in sight.

It was horrible, and I felt like I had travelled back to the time to just after my motorcycle accident.

Again I woke up after having only three hours of sleep. My head was pounding, and I felt sick to my stomach. I was shocked when I stared at the bathroom mirror. All the blood had drained from my face.

The room started to spin, and I quickly grabbed hold of the towel bar to steady myself. It felt like I was going to pass out.

Maybe the doctors missed something, I worried. *There must be something wrong with my brain.*

My stomach turned, and a cold sweat broke out on my back as I pictured myself all alone and going back to the hospital.

I stumbled to the bedroom and began to pace back and forth as if I was trying to wear out a trail in the carpet. My heart was pounding, and the sound of my breathing filled my ears. I had to clench my sweating fists to stop myself from chewing off my nails.

The silence of being alone made everything so much worse. This went on for the next hour before I couldn't take it anymore. Something was wrong, and I should probably call for an ambulance.

At that moment the phone rang. "Hello?" I whispered.

"Hi, Booman, how are you doing?" It was Jen. Instantly I felt a little better hearing her voice. I wished she were with me.

"Terrible," I groaned.

"What's wrong?" she asked, worried.

"I don't know, but it's really bad. I was just about to call for an ambulance."

"Why? What's happening?" cried Jen.

I paused to think and took a deep breath. "I'm so anxious, and it feels like my head is going to explode. I almost passed out because I'm so dizzy."

"Wait," she snapped. "This has happened to you before. I think I can help."

I didn't know what she was talking about.

"Remember a few years ago when we woke up in the middle of the night and you couldn't get back to sleep?"

"No." *How could I remember something that happened a few years ago?*

"It was the weekend when those teenagers woke us up. They threatened you, and we had to call the police."

I still couldn't remember what she was talking about. This was unusual, since I usually could remember experiences and events that were linked to strong emotions.

"The next day you were extremely tired and ended up having a panic attack. You thought you were dying back then as well," Jen recalled. "Go get your Wayne Dyer meditation CD."

"Why?" It amazed me that Jen could remember all these events in my life that I had completely forgotten about.

I had always enjoyed Dr. Dyer's books on spirituality, but I didn't know how this was going to help me now.

"Just get it," Jen urged. "You've forgotten."

It took me some time to find it, since I couldn't remember where my Dr. Dyer collection was.

"Good," she said when I finally found it. "Put it in the CD player and just listen. I bet you're going to give me five after this."

I pressed "play" and lay down on the bed, listening.

The music was soft and peaceful. Then Dr. Dyer's voice began: "*What I would like you to do first is get comfortable, close your eyes, be in any position that appeals to you...*"

A vague memory had been stirred.

I closed my eyes and listened, and my breathing slowed. So did my racing heart. For the next few minutes I lay and meditated in a peaceful state.

In ten minutes I had calmed down and felt much better. I felt like I could actually go to sleep.

I picked up the phone and listened to see if Jen was still there. "Boo," I said quietly.

"Yes, honey," said Jen.

"I give you five." I smiled. "I'm sorry, you are right. I feel so much better. Thanks a lot."

"I'm glad, Booman. Try to rest now."

Another miracle took place ... I fell asleep for fifteen minutes.

FYI: We have nicknames for each other. Jen is Boo and I am Booman :)

FYI # 2: Jen and I have an ongoing joke about the five most important words in a healthy relationship. For me these five words are... "I'm sorry, you are right." :)

DAY 5

Monday morning. I was alone and felt terrible. What was I going to do if the anxiety came back?

I wished Jen were there to help me.

After eating I went and grabbed my favourite Dr. Dyer book from the bookshelf. It was the one in which he had written about my story after he visited me in the ICU.

The phone rang. It was Jen.

"Are you doing okay?" she asked.

"Yeah, I'm okay," I replied.

I was very tired and had a really bad headache, but I didn't want to sound like a broken record saying the same thing over and over.

"Did you eat the breakfast I made for you?"

"Yeah, I just finished it. Delicious, thanks."

Jen had made me a smoothie filled with healthy ingredients.

"Good stuff, Booman. Remember what we learned about eating a nutritious breakfast?"

"Yes, I know, I know," I repeated. "Those who eat a nutritious breakfast help heal their brains."

"Uh-huh, that's right."

I was starting to realize that eating a good breakfast helped me deal with my constant fatigue.

"What are you going to do now?" she asked.

"I'm upstairs trying to read one of Dr. Dyer's books."

"Good idea. You should try to meditate. It might help you get some rest as well," she said softly. "Don't forget to call the neuropsychologist that your mom told you about."

"Okay," I said. "I'll do that after I meditate."

Fortunately, I was tired after meditating and chose to lie down and rest.

DAY 8

My day started off again with another phone call. I rolled out of bed and crawled to the phone.

"Hello?"

"You're still sleeping?"

I looked for my watch. "What time is it?"

"Sorry, honey. It's almost noon. I didn't expect you to still be in bed."

I yawned then cursed. "I'm not sleeping. Just lying in bed. Couldn't fall asleep again last night."

My nightly ritual of only getting three hours of sleep was really messing up my brain. Memory and concentration problems were made so much worse. Anxiety was always present, and I was always very grumpy and moody. It was torture. It didn't matter how tired I was, I could never go into a deep sleep. If I was lucky enough to fall asleep for a little bit during the day, I could forget about getting any sleep at night.

The sleep doctor at St. Michael's Hospital had told me the reason I was having sleep problems was that I had damaged my brain stem in my motorcycle accident, and my brain injury at work had exacerbated all my problems. The brain stem is an area of the brain involved in controlling many important life functions such as sleep, breathing, and heart rate. However, experience of fatigue after a traumatic brain injury varies greatly from person to person. Since everyone's brain is different, everyone will experience fatigue, as well as other symptoms, in a different way. When it comes to post-TBI fatigue, there are many factors that differ, such as level of severity and pervasiveness. Some people may experience fatigue all of the time, and others may only experience fatigue after mental and physical exertion. For me fatigue was with me all the time.

Most of my time was spent in bed or on the couch, hoping and praying that I might miraculously fall asleep.

"Hold on, wait one second," I said to Jen. "I'm just going to get a drink from the kitchen."

In the kitchen I found a note inside the fridge on my juice bottle. *Bon Appetit! Hi, love. I'm with you and thinking of you. I walked to the train while you were sleeping. Hope you had a better sleep.*

I walked back upstairs and picked up the phone. "I found your note. Thanks."

"Remember you have a doctor's appointment this afternoon," Jen said.

"Damn it," I said and then yawned. "I forgot."

"You don't have much time, Anthony," Jen urged. "Your dad's coming to get you in an hour. You better get ready."

Every day was a brand new day for me. I could never remember what had taken place the day before. Jen was my memory and my guide and would remind me what had happened the day before.

My dad had agreed to take me to my family doctor, since I needed a doctor's note to give to my work.

Two hours later, "How much longer?" I pleaded. My body was shaking, and I couldn't remember ever feeling so weak. The fatigue was torture.

"It's not much farther," said my dad.

I gazed around, frightened and scared. The other cars were moving so fast, it made my head spin.

I gripped the door handle and squeezed my eyes shut to keep the world from spinning.

I hoped this appointment wouldn't take long. All I wanted was to just get the doctor's note and be back home.

When I returned home, I was exhausted and lay on the couch feeling very sad and weak. It wasn't long before the tears were streaming down my face.

When is this hell going to end, I pleaded with myself.

I lay there alone with desperate thoughts. Life was not worth living if it was like this.

I sobbed myself to sleep — for only a few minutes.

Day 9

"Anthony, I have to get going now," whispered Jen.

I rubbed my eyes and fumbled for my watch. "What time is it?" I groaned. I felt so groggy, and my eyelids felt like they had weights on them.

"It's six thirty. You've been sleeping for almost seven hours!" said Jen with excitement. "You fell asleep almost right away after taking the new medication."

"What medication?"

"That one," said Jen, pointing.

My eyes widened in shock, and a sudden feeling of heaviness hit me when I saw the medication sitting right beside me on the bedside table.

"Where did I get this from?"

"From your doctor. You went there yesterday with your dad."

I stared remorsefully at the medication as a sickening feeling began to grow in the pit of my stomach. I had already used so much medication in the years following my motorcycle accident and didn't want that to continue. Depending on medication was not an option for me.

I struggled to remember the doctor's appointment. Nothing. I hated this. Forgetting everything. How could I go on with my brain that was obviously not working? Life was meaningless to me without memories. They were always hiding from me, and it was so much work to find them.

I wished I had remembered to use my iPhone® to record what the doctor had said. My iPhone was like my brain's external hard drive. It enabled me to remember everything that I recorded into it.

But it didn't matter now since I had forgotten. At least I got some more sleep. Although I knew I needed more sleep, I worried about the side effects and worried some more that I would become dependent on this medication.

If only I could deal with my brain injury without needing drugs.

"I only slept because of the medication," I complained to Jen. "It's not going to help my brain to heal."

I shook my head in frustration. "If I stop taking this medication, the same sleep problems will come back. I've already experienced this many times in the past."

Jen grabbed hold of my hand. "Love, I know it's difficult, but right now you need more sleep."

She leaned over to give me a kiss and then got up to leave. "Promise me you'll call the neuropsychologist your mom told you about."

I nodded.

"I'll call you from work."

Later that day I made an appointment with the neuropsychologist.

Day 10

I stepped on the GO train to head downtown. This was my first attempt at independence, but I was scared and unsure. Toronto was a huge city, and I was worried I would forget my way around and get lost. I had told Jen that I wanted to go by myself to my appointment with the neuropsychiatrist at St. Michael's Hospital. This was my first appointment with this doctor since my injury at school.

When I arrived at the hospital, the doctor walked me to his office.

The discussion began with me attempting to tell him about the brain injury I had sustained at school.

He was shocked and asked me about the problems I was having.

I stumbled over my words in embarrassment. "Problems sleeping ... I mean I can't ... because the anxiety ... just ... No, wait ... hold on!"

I stopped, flustered, and my cheeks were hot. I tried to clear my mind so that I could explain it clearly. Quickly, I thrust my hand into my pocket, feeling for my iPhone. Just holding it made me feel stronger.

"It's difficult to talk," I said as I looked out the window.

"Communication problems are common after a brain injury," the doctor said gently. "It's normal, and they are made a lot worse when you don't get the rest you need."

I nodded gently. "My sleep problems are so much worse."

The doctor continued. "Fatigue is something that most people have great difficulty with after a brain injury. It can drastically affect your life, and it will also affect your memory."

Slowly I nodded again. "Definitely, everything is so much harder now."

"I understand," he said softly. "It probably feels like you can only do half as much as you used to be able to do."

"Uh-huh," I said. "My brain gets tired so quickly now."

He nodded and pulled out a pad of paper. "I'm going to increase the dose of your medication."

He put down his pen. "If this doesn't work, we'll try a new medication."

He went on to warn me about the dangers of repetitive brain injuries and that rest was essential for me to heal my brain.

My head hung low as I dragged myself out of his office to go home.

Neurofeedback

~~~

Day 12

MY LEG JIGGLED NERVOUSLY AS I waited for the neuropsychologist, a psychologist who specialized in brain injuries — different than the psychiatrist, who was a medical doctor. I had arrived early hopeful with anticipation about getting some help with my sleep and anxiety problems.

When I had called to book my appointment, I learned that she used an alternative treatment that would help my brain heal itself. Healing my brain was the most important thing for me. Serious cognitive issues such as problems with my memory, concentration, and attention were still a big difficulty because of the sleep deprivation I experienced. Getting proper sleep is extremely important to help your brain learn and remember.

I had depended on sleep medications on and off for many years. The side effects were difficult for me to live with, and I was desperate to stop taking them. I was so tired of waking up feeling really groggy, tired, and sick to my stomach.

Hopefully this psychologist could help me stop taking them. There was no way I would have missed this appointment.

I sat and waited. Then waited some more as I skimmed over the health magazines. I thought about all the doctors I had seen for my problems.

The only solution was medication. Since my motorcycle accident, I had been prescribed an enormous number of medications for my problems. Medications for pain, depression, anxiety, anger, as well as my sleep problems. I also had to take medication after all the surgeries. Brain surgery, heart surgery, vascular surgery, lung surgery, plastic surgery, knee surgery... The list was endless.

Now here I was waiting to see another doctor.

But she wasn't a medical doctor like the others, and I was excited about the possibility of healing without having to pick up a prescription at a pharmacy.

After what seemed like forever, the psychologist finally appeared. She smiled and looked down at me.

"Anthony?"

I nodded.

She pointed toward her office. "Hi, sorry to keep you waiting. My office is just over here."

There were several pieces of furniture basking in the sunlight streaming in from the far window. A computer was on the desk sitting behind a comfy-looking couch. A few steps in front of the couch sat a video monitor reflecting the window behind the couch. The bookshelf behind the table at the side had lots of books about the brain. Too many to count.

I stared at the books and wondered if she knew that much about the brain.

Maybe she might be able to help me heal my brain.

"Please have a seat," she said and gestured toward the chair beside the table.

The seat had a soft cushion.

The psychologist looked professional in her dark trouser suit, and she beamed warmly. "Okay, why are you interested in neurofeedback?" she asked, pulling a chair up across from me while resting a notepad on her knee.

My thoughts and words stumbled over each other. I blushed and looked down at my hands. "My first brain injury was in 1997 because of a bad motorcycle accident," I said nervously.

She nodded slowly and looked at me thoughtfully.

"But only two weeks ago I had another brain injury at work."

"What work do you do?" she asked.

"I'm a teacher."

She nodded and continued to ask me questions. Her voice was soft and peaceful. "How did you sustain a brain injury at work?"

My thoughts froze and my cheeks started to burn. It was embarrassing, I couldn't find the right words to explain my thoughts. The words were on the tip of my tongue.

I looked up and took a deep breath. "It's difficult for me to speak."

She looked at me silently. It was a look that showed concern, understanding, and caring all at the same time.

Eventually I was able to tell her what had happened to me.

"You came to the right place," she said, smiling. "Neurofeedback can help you heal your brain."

I slowly nodded and smiled back at her.

She hadn't mentioned anything about having to take any medication.

"I have treated many people who have sustained a brain injury," she said. "Please feel free to ask any questions that you have."

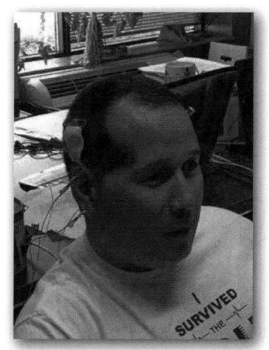

Anthony during a neurofeedback treatment session

I had a million questions. Probably more questions than she had books on her shelf. My brain was full of them, but I couldn't get them out.

After fifteen minutes of more questions, she guided me to the comfy sofa and said, "We'll start the neurofeedback with you sitting here."

I touched the little pads she attached to my head and looked at my reflection in the video monitor.

"What are these for?" I asked.

"They're brain wave sensors," she said.

She was sitting right behind me, doing something at her computer.

"In neurofeedback we need to see what your brain waves are doing in order to make changes to your brain wave pattern."

"Huh?"

I didn't understand.

"Everyone has brain waves," she continued. "It's the electrical activity coming from the brain."

"Uh-huh," I said, trying to commit to memory what she was saying.

"You see, the brain has the ability to self-correct and make changes to itself when it is given the right information. Neurofeedback is like training for your brain! This program will provide your brain with the information it needs to make its own adjustments. It's a drug-free brain exercise that helps to change an unhealthy brainwave pattern into a healthy one."

My ears perked up, and my heart started beating a little faster when I heard her say "drug-free."

"You are going to hear some music during the session. When your brain is functioning smoothly, the music will play smoothly and in time with the patterns you'll see on the video screen. But when the music crackles and gets interrupted, this is a signal telling your brain that it is not working efficiently."

I nodded but quickly stopped because it made my head hurt. "This sounds like a teacher pointing out their students' mistakes and reminding them when to make some changes."

"Exactly," said the psychologist, sounding quite pleased. "Your brain learns when it's stuck, and with practice your brain improves and works more effectively."

I was anxious to start, wondering what it was going to feel like.

"Okay, let's start now," she said, "but first, I need to do a check on your brain waves. Eyes open. No talking or moving for thirty seconds."

It was difficult to sit still. I was nervous but tried to remain calm and hopeful. Thoughts were racing through my brain.

What if it doesn't work for me?

My forehead wrinkled.

What if my brain is too damaged?

I bit my lip and stared at the floor.

Can she see my thoughts on her computer?

I had to stop myself from thinking.

What if she *could* tell what I was thinking? Maybe the wires attached to my head would send my thoughts to her computer, and then she would know.

At that moment a pattern of coloured bars appeared on the video monitor. Soft and peaceful music started to play. It was relaxing.

I listened and stared at the bars on the screen, which seemed to move in time with the music. Suddenly the music paused and there was a crackling sound. It sounded like TV static.

I leaned forward. My heart was beating fast as I looked closely at the bars on the screen.

This must be that crackling sound she was talking about. What is wrong, and why has the music paused? What is my brain doing right now?

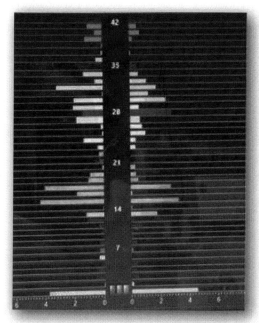

The video screen during neurofeedback

I wondered what was happening.

Can she tell that there is something wrong with my brain?

The coloured bars continued to move on the video monitor.

It was like someone had turned on a switch to start the crackling noise. It stopped soon after it started, almost as if the switch had been turned off.

This pattern of the music, frequently interrupted by the crackling sound, continued for the next forty-five minutes.

By the time the music stopped playing, I felt very calm and at peace and was ready for sleep. Something had happened. My brain felt different — like it was learning and making changes to itself.

"Okay, let's do a quick check before we finish," said the psychologist. "Keep your eyes open. No talking or moving for thirty seconds."

She repeated this with my eyes closed.

Once finished, she removed the sensors and cleaned up the sticky paste that held the electrodes to my head.

Later that night, I felt a sense of peace and serenity I hadn't ever experienced before.

Day 13

"You slept a long time," said Jen.

I was reading in bed, and Jen was getting ready for work.

I smiled when I looked at the clock. It was 6:00 a.m.

"I know," I replied. "Something feels different." I stopped moving and thought hard.

"I feel stronger, but I still have a headache," I grumbled. "It's probably because of the medication."

"Still, that's a great improvement," said Jen excitedly. Her eyes sparkled. "You fell asleep by ten last night." She had broken into a wide grin.

"Yeah." I nodded. "And I slept straight until 4:00 a.m.!"

"That's a six-hour sleep!" Jen almost shouted. "You've never had that before."

I wanted to stop taking my medication, but the psychologist had told me that I should never stop taking medication cold turkey. It was important for me to continue to take the medication until I knew the treatment was helping me.

Having a restorative sleep got me hooked on neurofeedback. I knew that the improvement in my sleep wasn't because of the medication, since I had never felt like this before.

After taking sleep medication, I always woke up feeling drugged and extremely groggy. This led to serious memory lapses throughout the day. I hated feeling like this, making it an easy decision to continue with neurofeedback, and in time I eventually weaned myself off all medication.

DAY 23

I had just finished another neurofeedback session and again felt very calm. At the end of the session, I was feeling so good that I didn't want it to end.

"How was that?" asked the psychologist.

"It was great." I smiled. "It feels like my brain is beginning to heal."

"Wonderful," she replied. "The effects of your brain injury will be reduced by this brain training." She finished wiping off the remaining electrode paste. "I want you to keep paying attention and noticing anything that is new, different, or missing,"

At home I thought about what she had said. Things were improving for me. The anxiety that was a result of my poor sleep was decreasing. This had a positive effect on the depression I was experiencing. I was starting to feel happier and less burdened with depressed thoughts.

All these changes were most certainly related to the improvement in my sleep.

If things continued to improve for me, I would be able to return to work soon. This had been a long break, and I didn't have any more sick days. The insurance company had refused to accept my claim for an extended sick leave because of my brain injury. They said my current problems were because of a pre-existing injury, so I did not qualify for any worker's compensation.

The financial implications of continuing to stay on sick leave worried me.

I needed some reassurance that I was getting better, especially since Jen and I had already made plans to travel to Australia during the Christmas holidays. We were going to visit my grandmother in Tasmania, as she had just celebrated her 102nd birthday. But the twenty-four-hour travel time with multiple flights scared me.

Would I be able to handle it? Would the anxiety take control of me? How would this travel affect my sleep?

The self-doubt and questions were unending. If only I had proof that I was getting stronger. Going back to work and succeeding would be great for my self-confidence.

But would it be possible for me to go back to work before the Christmas holidays?

It would be best to ask the psychologist.

Day 30

The psychologist looked up, smiling, when I walked into her office. She was typing away at her computer and seemed glad to see me. "Hi Anthony," she said. "We'll get started in a minute."

I sat in my regular spot on the comfy couch with the video monitor right in front of me.

It wasn't long before she was beside me, attaching the electrodes to my head. "There, you're all connected now. Let's do a check first," she said.

After the check, I carefully turned around to her, making sure I didn't pull off any of the electrodes. "I'd like to ask you something at the end of the session."

She nodded. "That's fine."

When the session was over and I was free from the wires, she pulled up a chair in front of me. "Okay, what is it that you wanted to talk about?"

"Next week is the last week of school before the Christmas holidays." I looked down at my iPhone, holding it firmly. "During the Christmas holidays we are travelling to Australia. I need to feel more confident that I am stronger and will be able to handle this long trip."

I stopped to think. Then I thought some more. The past month had felt like an eternity. The last time I had been off work for longer than a few days was sixteen years ago when I had my motorcycle accident, which, by the way, was what the insurance company considered my pre-existing injury!

"Damn it," I cursed, pushing my iPhone back into my pocket. "I forgot what I was talking about."

"You were talking about your upcoming Christmas holidays," the psychologist reminded me.

"Oh, yeah," I said, shaking my head. "Since this is the last week before Christmas holidays, I think this would be a good week for me to return to work."

I looked at her, almost pleading for her approval. "I won't be too stressed," I continued. "Before the holidays it is a less hectic schedule in the classroom."

She was nodding and looked like she was thinking. "When I first saw you almost three weeks ago, you were having a lot more difficulties than you are having now. The neurofeedback has definitely been very helpful to you. I think you will be able to handle this, if you take things slowly."

I nodded.

"Treat everything like it's an experiment," she continued. "If the experiment doesn't work out as you want it to, then make some changes and try the experiment again. And make sure you see me for a session after your first day."

I listened carefully, hoping I would remember what she said.

My memory problems worried me a lot. I hoped I would be able to find a way to cope with them when I was back at school. They were almost as bad as during the early stages after my motorcycle accident.

DAY 37

It was my first day back at school after my brain injury. I gripped the steering wheel as I drove. My heart was pounding. I was trying not to panic. This was my first time driving since my injury, and I was driving by myself. I had to get to school, otherwise I'd have to take another sick day.

It was six thirty in the morning, and I still had a lot to do before class started. My hands tightened around the steering wheel as I struggled to remember the names of my students.

How am I going to manage at school?

The other cars raced by me as I drove very carefully. Sweat trickled down my neck. The anxiety was almost crippling.

I moved closer to the steering wheel, staring intently at the road and the surroundings. I held my breath and tried to keep myself from moving unnecessarily. I didn't want the dizziness to come back. All the other cars seemed to be so close to me, almost like they were touching my car. My hands were almost numb from gripping the steering wheel so hard. The thought of having another accident was terrifying.

Peering through the front window, I could make out the park filled with trees just in front of the school.

I pulled into the parking lot and breathed deeply. "Made it." I breathed a loud sigh of relief.

The school was empty, and my footsteps echoed in the barren hallways. It was a disaster for me when I walked into my classroom.

"Oh, come on!" I cursed. I was so angry that my classroom had been re-organized. It felt like I was walking into a completely different classroom. My desk had been re-organized, with everything moved. It got worse; all my books and teaching supplies had been moved to different locations around the classroom.

I couldn't work like this. Everything in my class had a special spot to help me remember where they were. Whenever I needed something, I would go to its special spot, and it would be there. But now I had no idea where anything was. The next hour was spent finding everything and moving it back to its proper location.

After some time in my classroom, I heard footsteps in the hall. The footsteps were coming closer and closer.

Suddenly a young woman appeared in the door. Her face had a big smile, and her eyes were filled with happiness.

"Tanya," I called out and walked over to give her a hug.

"I heard that you might be coming back today." She beamed, resting her bag on a desk. "Are you re-organizing your class ?" she asked as she glanced around.

"No," I said wearily. "Someone moved all of my stuff, so I'm just putting everything back where I need it to be."

"Would you like help?" she asked, the concern evident in her voice.

I shook my head and anxiously looked at the clock. "No thanks. I have to get back to work. Lots to do before school starts."

The rest of the day went fine, with the exception of the memory problems I experienced.

I was very pleased, as my students were unusually supportive and didn't pay attention to any memory lapses that I had. They were unusually well behaved. Everything went great.

At the end of the school day I was exhausted. My eyelids were heavy, and I struggled to stay awake as I pulled out of the parking lot. I was off to my neurofeedback appointment. Shaking my head to wake myself, I drove off slowly and carefully. Almost immediately, I felt woozy and had to squint to see the signs on the road. I felt helpless and scared, and then the anxiety came back. Cold sweat, nausea, and a racing heart all coursed through my veins. My knuckles turned white as I gripped the steering wheel. It didn't feel like I was moving as the other cars raced past.

After only a few minutes I had to pull over to the side of the road. There was not much of a shoulder, but luckily I managed to find a driveway to pull into.

It felt like I was going to die. The cold air woke me up a bit as I walked around the car, trying to clear my head.

For the next twenty minutes I continued going around and around the car until I felt strong enough to drive.

Once at my appointment, I dragged myself into the clinic bathroom. I turned on the faucet and splashed cold water on my face. My reflection showed a tired, anxious man with a look of sorrow in his eyes.

After the neurofeedback, a miracle happened. The drive home was quick and easy, without any strain or anxiety.

The next morning I woke up without any difficulty. My head wasn't hurting, and I wasn't dizzy. I looked around and felt so pleased that the room was not spinning. Jen was already up and smiling at me as she walked over.

"You did it."

"What?"

"You had another six-hour sleep."

I looked at the clock and tried to remember my sleep. "You're right, and I didn't even wake up in the middle of the night."

Days went by, and then weeks. The Christmas holidays in Australia were a lot of fun. It was great to see my grandmother and celebrate her birthday.

I was amazed at how strong she was and then realized that I had inherited much strength from her.

The flights to Australia and back were very long and tiring. Once back in Canada, my sleep, fatigue, and anxiety problems intensified due to the jet lag.

DAY 54

The days back at school were very difficult since I wasn't going for neurofeedback any more. The sleep and anxiety problems had returned.

I found it very difficult to remember even the simplest information, as my brain was always in a fog. The fatigue also led to problems with attention and concentration.

SCIENCE NOTES

The following information came from several sources, as outlined in the references at the end of this book. Neurofeedback is a very beneficial treatment for brain injuries. It is also called EEG biofeedback because it is based on brain electrical activity, the electroencephalogram (EEG).

It is a direct training of brain function, by which the brain learns to function more efficiently. It is the process of training the brain to learn to modify or control brainwave activity through auditory and visual feedback. Neurofeedback is a noninvasive method of creating a balance within the central nervous system, and it is 100% safe, gentle, and painless.

The brain is a neuroplastic organ capable of changing its own pathways and structure. Because it is amazingly adaptable, it can easily learn to make adjustments to improve its own performance.

During a neurofeedback session, the central nervous system is given comprehensive information in "real time" about its behaviour. That information will help the brain restore its optimal functioning. It's as if you are holding a mirror to your brain. Once you see your reflection, you might want to adjust yourself to attain the desired appearance; maybe this means that you change the way that you are standing or you change your hair, etc. The mirror provides the feedback so you can make the desired adjustments. The brain works in a similar way.

When given the right information, the brain can make changes to the way that it works. During a neurofeedback session, the brain is provided with the necessary information in order for it to make its own adjustments.

This "brain training" does not require a person to consciously attain any specific mental state, since the training happens unconsciously through the auditory and visual feedback.

Participants sit quietly, listening to soothing music during a neurofeedback session. Brief interruptions in the music provide feedback to the brain. Visual feedback can also be delivered to the participant. The participant does not need to respond in any active way to the feedback or even attend to it consciously, because the brain, a complex adaptive system, uses the feedback for its own process of self-organization without reliance on conscious intervention.

Day 62

The holidays had passed, and I had settled into a familiar routine at school, which made it easier for me to remember what I needed to do.

Day 66

The weekend came, and I sat in the kitchen drinking my decaf coffee. I had become obsessive about avoiding all caffeine to ensure that my sleep would not be affected.

I was thinking about the jobs I had to do. Clean the car, wash the dishes, organize the storage room. The list felt endless, yet I had promised Jen I would get these jobs done. But I didn't have the motivation to get started. It was too much for my brain to think about. Doing it seemed almost impossible.

Fatigue, a familiar feeling, overtook me. I headed for the bedroom to lie down. If I meditated, just maybe I might be lucky enough to fall asleep. Meditating and resting in bed had become a necessity. Where had my motivation gone? Before my brain injuries I used to be a person full of energy, with dreams of going to the Olympics. Now it was such an effort just to get up and get dressed. I lay on the bed and meditated. Lucky for me, I fell asleep. This was good, even if it was only for a few minutes.

When I awoke, the familiar feelings of fatigue were there ... a headache, nausea, and an overall body ache.

I was angry at the brain injuries I had sustained. I didn't know why this had to happen to me and was unsure of what would happen with my teaching career.

There was a mixture of fatigue, anxiety, helplessness, and fear for the future that blended in with all the other emotions.

Damn it, I thought. *Why me*!

I lay back down on the bed and looked at my watch.

Three thirty. I hadn't done anything. I was always so tired. Jen would be home from her appointment soon.

... THE GYM ?

When Jen came home, she called up from the front door. "Honey, why don't we go check out that new gym?" I was lying in bed, and the last thing I wanted was to check out some gym.

"No!," I shouted down to her. "I'm trying to rest."

"But you said that we should exercise more in the new year."

"Not now, I'm too tired!"

"Anthony," Jen's voice was getting closer. "You said that when you are able to work out, it helps you feel a little better. But you haven't done much in a while."

"You wouldn't be doing anything either if you didn't get any sleep." I shouted. My angry outbursts were happening more frequently. It didn't matter what someone else did … I was always upset. I hated feeling like this all the time.

Jen walked into the bedroom and knelt down beside the bed. "I know it is very difficult for you. I don't know how you do it. I know I couldn't do it."

She reached over and lifted my chin to look directly at me. "Don't worry, we'll face this together. Remember, TEAAM."

She was always saying that and had added the extra A into the spelling of TEAAM to stand for our last name, Aquan-Assee.

Day 73

The following week on Saturday, we were getting ready to go to the new gym that had opened up near us. Jen was smiling suspiciously as she did up her shoes.

"I hope you like the trainer I picked for us."

My stomach suddenly dropped; I felt like it had just been kicked. "What do you mean a trainer that you picked for us," I shouted.

"Well, it was a secret." She giggled. "I went there and arranged for a trainer to train both of us."

"I don't need a trainer," I shouted. I was shocked that she had gone behind my back and arranged this. "I could be a trainer if I wanted to," I blurted. "Are you going for the saint of the year award?"

I wished that I had not said that as soon as the words left my lips.

She just looked at me with sadness in her eyes.

"Sorry," I said. "I didn't mean to sound so mean. I'm just really tired."

"You're always tired."

I went upstairs and lay down on the bed. My jaw clenched in frustration.

What's my problem? I thought. *Why am I always losing control?*

Before my motorcycle accident, I had been in amazing shape and had competed very passionately in judo as well as in body-building. My judo sensei was the North American Heavyweight Judo Champion, and he was my main competitor at the club. Whenever I competed against him, I always did very well. It had been my dream to represent Canada in judo at the 2000 Olympics in Sydney, Australia, and I had his full support and encouragement to go after my dreams. So in the months prior to my accident, I had been training very hard, hoping to compete in the Canadian National Judo Championships. If I did well in this tournament, maybe, just maybe, I might have had a chance to go to the Olympics. But then I had my motorcycle accident and lost this dream forever.

Ha! Me need a trainer. The next hour was spent lying on the bed in a mixed state of fatigue, anxiety, and insecurity.

Working out had always been a big part of my life, and I never needed anyone to help me. Now here my wife was telling me that a trainer would be good to push me and give me some motivation.

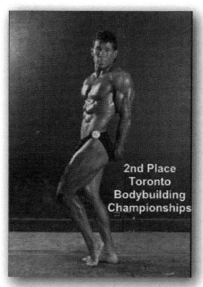

Second place in the Toronto Body-Building Championships (1994)

I hadn't had a neurofeedback session in a few weeks, and it was beginning to show. My mind was flooded with thoughts of the past and worries for my future. I felt like I was trapped in a nightmare, and I couldn't escape it. Anxiety and fatigue screamed at me from every part of my body. The fatigue and emotional pain fed off each other and led to a sense of hopelessness. I had to do something to put an end to this hell I was living.

Jen came over and gently squeezed my hand. "Honey, it's getting late. We have to get going to the gym."

I rolled over and turned away from her. "I don't feel like exercising and definitely not with a trainer."

She squeezed my hand some more. "Exercise will help with the fatigue. And think about this," she paused and pointed at my head, "exercising will get more oxygen pumped to your brain. This will improve your thinking, and it will help your brain to heal itself. Think how good you will feel when your brain begins to heal itself."

I was embarrassed. Jen was right.

It really didn't matter that a trainer was going to help me. They could probably help make my road to recovery a smooth one. If this could help my brain heal, this was all that mattered.

I turned to Jen. "I'm sorry, honey, you are right."

Jen smiled. "I only want the best for you."

"Let's get going." I half grinned. "We don't want to be late."

Cranial Electrotherapy Stimulation (CES)

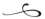

Day 77

"CLASS MEETING," I ANNOUNCED TO the afternoon gym class. I sat in a chair with all the kids sitting in a circle around me.

"It looks like you all have earned enough points to choose your favourite gym activity."

"Yeah!" the kids screamed, throwing their arms in the air. They stood up, full of excitement, cheering and clapping.

"Let's have a game of soccer," cried Chris. He was the most popular kid in the class but definitely not the best athlete. The kids jumped forward, and teams were chosen. Chris and Steven were the captains. They did rock, paper, scissors for the first pick. Chris won. They went on to choose their teams.

Once the game began, Chris never stopped running.

He ran up and down the gym, chasing after the ball, but was rarely able to catch up to it. Chris would kick wildly as soon as he got within ten feet of the ball, but someone else would kick it first. Most of the time he ended up kicking the other players instead of kicking the ball. He almost kicked me, even though I was standing just outside the red line.

Near the end of the game, Chris found himself alone with the ball and on a breakaway to the net. The whistles and shouts of the other players urged him on. He kicked the ball hard into the air, but instead of going straight, the ball veered off to the side. Before I could step out of danger, the ball smashed me in the head.

I blacked out and fell face-first to the floor. The kids ran over to me. "Mr. A, are you okay?" they shrieked. Some time went by before my eyes opened. I rolled over and tried to focus.

My head and face throbbed with a sharp pain. I felt something trickling from my nose. When I wiped it, my hand was covered in blood.

The students gasped, and I could see the fear and concern in their eyes.

"Get the principal," I whispered. My body was shaking, and I felt very weak. The students helped me to sit up. I gazed around, but the room was spinning.

I grasped my head to ease the pain and remained on the gym floor.

The principal arrived and helped me get upstairs to the main office.

Jen was horrified when the office called her.

"What happened?" she shouted. I wasn't even holding the phone, but I could hear her voice.

Her eyes were red with tears by the time she came to my school to pick me up.

Even before we arrived at the hospital, I knew that I had sustained another brain injury. A short time later, the hospital ER doctor confirmed another horrible nightmare.

After this, all the problems I was experiencing got so much worse. I felt hopelessly inept and bewildered by my problems.

My thinking was painfully slow, and I was easily confused. Severe headaches and dizziness kept my mind locked in a world of isolation. It felt as if my world was spinning out of control. My mind was rigid, and thinking became limited; I couldn't think beyond the moment. Even if I were hit with a stroke of insight, I would never remember it. Extreme anxiety and other strong emotions tormented me all the time. This certainly was made far worse with the terrible sleep I got every night.

DAY 79

I arrived at the psychologist's office hoping to get an appointment with her, even though I had not called for one. Things were not improving, so I just got Jen to drop me off.

She was sitting at her desk in front of her computer.

I knocked on her door and walked in when she waved me in. Once inside, I perched nervously on the edge of the seat by her desk.

Stay calm. She can help, I told myself.

But inside I was screaming with anxiety.

She looked up from her computer. Her forehead was wrinkled, and she stared at me in surprise.

"Why are you here?" she asked.

I sighed. "I'm sorry I didn't call."

She nodded and quickly glanced at the door. "What's wrong?"

I nodded but quickly stopped. My head was hurting too much. "I had another brain injury a few days ago."

Her eyes widened, and she quickly stood up. "What happened?" she asked.

I stood there trying to gather my thoughts.

For the next little while I told her about the soccer game and about the soccer ball hitting me; how I was knocked out in front of my students; how I had to go to the hospital again; how I had to have another CAT scan; how the doctor told me that I had sustained another brain injury; how I had been told that I was to stay off work until I had been cleared by my family doctor; and that the only person I knew who could help me now was her. It was obvious that I was close to breaking down, so she stepped forward and guided me to the comfy couch.

It was a struggle when I tried to tell her the problems I was having. "Sleep is terrible, and so is the anxiety. Wait! Hold on!" My brain was stuck and stopped working. My words froze, and I forgot what I was talking about.

I looked down and sighed. My head was shaking in frustration. "Sorry," I whispered.

I reached inside my pocket, feeling for my iPhone.

The psychologist reached over to pat my arm. "This probably feels like a never-ending battle," she said softly as she finished connecting the wires to my scalp.

"Uh-huh," I said. "My brain is so messed up now."

She nodded. "Just sit back and relax."

The soft, peaceful music began to play, and the coloured bars appeared on the video monitor.

Almost immediately I felt relaxed. Things felt so much better when the treatment was over.

"Can I come again next week?" I asked hopefully.

"Well..." She paused and then walked back to her desk. "I'm not sure about my schedule..." she continued with a slight break in her voice. "You'll have to call me next week." She fumbled through her desk drawer. "Just in case we won't be able to do a session next week, I want you to borrow my CES device once I find it."

I didn't understand what she was talking about. "Huh? What's a CES device? Is it the same as neurofeedback?"

She shook her head. "No. One second, and I'll show you what I have."

She continued searching through her desk drawer. "CES is short for Cranial Electrotherapy Stimulation. This is a treatment for when you have problems with sleep, anxiety, and depression. All the problems you are currently experiencing. It is a small, handheld device about the size of a smartphone that sends a mild electrical current to the brain using ear clip electrodes."

She closed the drawer and opened the bottom one. "Ah-ha, here it is," she declared.

She opened the box and pulled out the device and the instructions. She then showed me how to attach the clip electrodes to my ears and how to turn it on.

"Here." She placed the box in my hand. "Take this home and give it a try. Let me know if it helps."

Just then there was a knock at the door and a face peered in through the window. She looked over and held up her hand.

"Give me five minutes." She turned back to me. "I'm really sorry, Anthony, but I have to see my patient. Please call me next week and see if there is space for a treatment session. This should help you in the meantime. Now go try this out."

When I left, I was worried that this device was going to shock my brain, just as in electroshock therapy (ECT) to treat depression. It reassured me after I read the instructions and learned that ECT uses a steady, strong electrical current applied directly to the scalp, whereas the CES device applies a pulsing current that is over a thousand times weaker to the earlobes.

I used the device for twenty minutes before I went to bed that night. After I had attached the ear clips, I felt a tingling sensation in my earlobes. This was a peculiar feeling, but the instructions had stated this was normal. I was able to turn the adjustment dial to change the settings until the sensation was comfortable. After twenty minutes, my mind was clear and more alert, and I felt very relaxed. I fell asleep shortly after using it. When I awoke, I was amazed to see that I had been able to get a five-and-a-half-hour sleep. This helped me so much and was almost as good as a neurofeedback session.

The same thing took place the following day.

The sleep benefits continued whenever I used this device. This in turn helped to reduce the anxiety and depression I was experiencing as my sleep improved. The psychologist continued to let me use her CES device until I purchased my own.

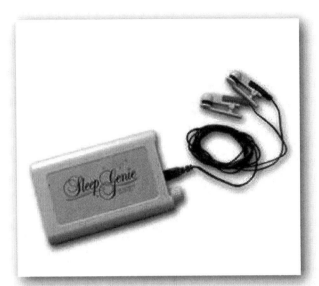

Cranial Electrotherapy Stimulation with the Sleep Genie

SCIENCE NOTES

The following information came from several sources, as outlined in the references at the end of this book.

Cranial Electrotherapy Stimulation (CES) is a medical treatment designed in the USSR to treat sleep disorders, hence its original name, "electrosleep." Eventually the name was changed to cranial electrotherapy stimulation after it was available in the United States for treating anxiety and depression, as well as sleep.

This device is similar in appearance to a TENS device (Transcutaneous Electrical Nerve Stimulators) used for pain relief. However, a CES device produces a much milder electric current with electric pulses that can be adjusted depending on the desired treatment effect.

CES devices are painless and noninvasive brain stimulators. Other biomedical electronics, such as deep brain stimulating electrodes (used to treat seizures and hand tremors related to Parkinson's disease) and heart pacemakers are invasive and require surgical implantation.

Many brain problems occur because the brain's nerve cells, or neurons, are not firing properly. This can lead to low levels of important neurotransmitters such as serotonin, norepinephrine, and dopamine. These brain chemicals are necessary to communicate information throughout our brain and body.

The CES device is used to combat problems with low levels of these neurotransmitters, which are associated with depression and anxiety.

Once the small electric current in the CES device stimulates the brain, neurons are triggered to increase the release of serotonin, norepinephrine, and dopamine. Neurons are also triggered to release endorphins, which block the sensation of pain and lead to a sense of well-being. It has been reported that the CES device causes changes to the blood flow in the brain, helping to bring the brain's electrochemistry back into balance.

The nervous system works through both chemical and electrical signals. With CES technology, treatment based on the body's extensive electrical fields has emerged as a viable alternative to drugs and surgery.

When properly used, cranial electrotherapy stimulation can alleviate anxiety, depression, and/or insomnia, and improve the quality of your life.

The Cranial Electrotherapy Stimulator had improved my sleep, and I was getting about five hours of sleep each night. This was an improvement from the three hours I was getting after the brain injuries I sustained at school. But it wasn't enough, and I was always tired. This affected every part of my life. I still had hope that something more could be done. My elusive search for a "cure-all" treatment led me to a sleep specialist who also had a specialty in neuroscience.

Laser Therapy

"YOU HAVE A SLEEP DISORDER with an absence of deep sleep. Come back and see me after you have tried homeopathy and laser therapy."

The doctor was standing beside her desk. On the wall hung her medical degree from the University of Toronto and her certificates in neuroscience and sleep medicine from Stanford University.

"Huh?" My eyebrows came together in confusion.

I was familiar with homeopathy but not laser therapy. "What's laser therapy?"

"Here." She handed me a pamphlet on laser therapy. "Take this home to read." She took off her stethoscope. "Laser therapy uses light energy to heal your body. It's a good treatment for sleep problems."

"Is it safe ?" My forehead wrinkled.

"Absolutely," said the doctor. "Very safe. Better for you than all those sleep medications you've been on. The light energy from the laser is absorbed by the cells, which results in a natural way of healing."

"Okay, I think. Umm, I just never heard about this before."

I shook my head in disbelief. A doctor had never suggested this to me before.

"Before I came to see you, I saw five other sleep doctors and had sleep assessments with all of them, but none of them ever mentioned this to me."

She smiled at me. "That's because I'm different. I'm not into pushing pills. You should also sign up for my meditation group."

I smiled and looked down at the pamphlet. If only I had known about this doctor years ago.

My family doctor had referred me to see this sleep specialist when the insurance money ran out for the neurofeedback sessions. He figured she would be ideal, since she had training in neuroscience as well as psychiatry. I had come here knowing that she was different. It pleased me even more when I learned just how different she really was.

"Where do I go for laser therapy ?" I asked.

She pointed at the pamphlet. "It tells you in there, and there's a map on the back. The clinic is run by a doctor who used to be a surgeon. His name is Dr. Kahn."

We talked some more, and I had a big smile on my face when I learned that her priority was on integrating mind/body medicine with her patients to help them improve their health. Maybe she could help me taper off the medications.

Searching for health and wholeness in my life was very important to me, so I agreed to make another appointment with her after trying out laser therapy.

The first laser therapy treatment session was great. At first I thought that I was going to feel some heat when the laser therapist placed the laser across the back of my neck. But there was no heat. The therapist told me that "hot" lasers are high-intensity and can burn through flesh. Instead, she placed a low-intensity laser, or an array of superluminous diodes, across the back of my neck. She said this area was close to my brain stem, the area of the brain that regulates sleep, so they wanted to make sure this area was targeted by the laser.

I was told that the therapists would begin by treating the neck and base of the skull first. The brain stem (which extends downward through the base of the skull) connects to the motor and sensory parts of the brain that communicate with the rest of the body. It also regulates the central nervous system and is responsible for vital functions such as sleep regulation, breathing, heart rate, blood pressure, and consciousness. Treating these areas would allow the neck and the brain to receive blood flow and restore nerve connections, while also treating the injured tissue.

The forty-five-minute session was very relaxing. During the treatment I fell into a light sleep and had one of those dreams where I was half asleep and half awake.

The session was amazing, and afterward I felt relaxed and very refreshed. My brain was clear and alert.

The next morning, I was amazed when I saw that I had been able to get a six-hour sleep that night and did not have any grogginess when I awoke. I also could remember dreaming during the night. Since my motorcycle accident, this had never happened to me, even when I was taking sleep medication.

At future treatment sessions I learned that laser therapy would be good for my injured knee as well as for my brain. I had broken my knee in my motorcycle accident and lived with constant knee pain, which made walking difficult. From then on, the laser therapy treatment sessions focused both on my injured knee as well as my brain. The therapists would place an array of super luminous diodes across the back of my neck as well and simultaneously across my knee.

The results were outstanding. After my first dual combination treatment session, my knee felt considerably better, and I was tired enough to go home and have a nap.

Laser therapy treatment sessions continued for the next few months.

My experiences with the therapy were extremely positive for my sleep and cognitive problems. After a therapy session I no longer felt any brain fog, and my memory improved greatly. This was also very positive for my knee and significantly reduced my knee pain. As the treatment sessions continued, I usually got about six hours of sleep.

After I discovered laser therapy, my condition improved so much that I was able to resume my daily workouts as well as my daily walks lasting thirty minutes or more.

I began to think that this was the "cure-all" treatment I had been searching for.

Science Notes

The following information came from several sources, as outlined in the references at the end of this book.

Low Intensity Laser Therapy (LILT) is the use of light from a low-intensity laser diode or an array of superluminous diodes to eliminate pain, accelerate healing, and decrease inflammation. It is nontoxic and is an effective and noninvasive way to repair a damaged brain and an injured body. Laser therapy can be used to improve sleep, eliminate pain, stimulate the immune system, and restore the normal range of motion in one's body.

Researchers have found that laser light at a specific wavelength can penetrate the skull and increase blood flow in the brain. It also stimulates the mitochondria, which produces energy in the cell in the form of a energy molecule called ATP. When the mitochondria are stimulated by the light energy, more ATP is produced, thus increasing the energy molecules available to the cell. This causes complex biochemical processes that result in the restoration of normal cell structure and function.

The treatment is very safe, while promoting natural healing, and has no adverse side effects. It is highly effective in treating brain injuries, musculoskeletal conditions, arthritis, sports injuries, wound healing, and a wide range of dermatological conditions.

Laser therapy gets to the root of a problem and offers lasting solutions, as opposed to other therapies, many of which only mask the perception of pain or modulate symptoms.

Kangen Water®

I SAT EXCITED, TAPPING MY fingers to the music that was playing.

The Apple Store was packed, and the workshop was going to start soon. Paul, the trainer, was playing some music on his computer.

"Your music sounds great," I said. "What's the CD?"

Paul shook his head. "It's not a CD, it's from GarageBand."

"Seriously, who helped you make this?" I was amazed and hoped that I would learn how to do this.

"No one," said Paul smiling. "I made this music by myself. You are going to learn how to do this as well."

I was very excited and couldn't wait to learn how to do this. I loved playing my guitar and spent many sleepless nights strumming away, wishing I had a band to jam with. Now if I could learn this, I could be my own band and wouldn't need anyone else.

Just then an older woman sat down at the table. "Hi there," she said, smiling.

I was surprised to see her, as I was expecting younger guys to be at the workshop.

"Hi," I replied.

Paul began the workshop by sharing some other songs he had created.

The workshop was amazing. We learned how to record an instrument and then how to edit the music using GarageBand.

We were making music by ourselves and not having to rely on anyone else.

Time went quickly, and we learned a lot. By the end of the workshop my brain was full and too tired to remember any more information.

As I put away my computer, I overheard the older woman, Ruth, telling another woman that her sister had recently been diagnosed with cancer.

I immediately felt empathy for her, as my mother-in-law had also recently gone through a very difficult battle with cancer.

Turning to her, I expressed my condolences. "I'm sorry to hear about this."

She smiled. "Thanks. Learning like this is a great way for me to forget about my health problems."

"No kidding," I replied, nodding. "I feel the same as you." I was surprised that someone shared my feelings. I wondered what health challenges she faced. The look on my face must have told her what I was thinking.

"I have lived with osteoporosis for many years. But two years ago my health problems improved greatly when I started drinking Kangen Water®."

"What's that?" I asked.

"Kangen Water® is alkaline water, a healthier form of water."

I reached for my iPhone so I could record the name.

Alkaline water, I thought. *This sounds natural. I wonder if it could help me.*

"Here is my card," I said. "Can you please email me the information about this water?"

Later that night I received an email from her.

Her message immediately caught my attention, as it contained interesting information. This included some testimonials about Kangen Water® from medical doctors. She told me I could try it for free on a trial basis at a health food store close to me. That was the motivation I needed to try out this Kangen Water®.

I had been off all medications for months now but I was still searching for that "cure-all" treatment. Maybe this might be the one and I could use it in the comfort of my own home.

It was snowing and the driving conditions weren't great, but I was determined to go to the health food store that Ruth had told me about to try out this water. When I walked in, a man stood in the middle of the store stocking the shelves.

"Hi," he said.

"Hi," I replied. "I was told that I would be able to try some Kangen Water® here."

He smiled and walked behind the counter. "Yes, of course," he said. "Who told you this?"

"I can't remember her name, but I met her at the Apple Store."

"Ah, yes. You must be Anthony."

I nodded, wondering how he knew my name.

He placed a yellow folder on the countertop.

"I'm Jeff. Ruth called me and told me about you. She said that she met you at the Apple Store and that you might be coming here to learn more about it."

I nodded again.

He showed me a newspaper article with a picture of a Japanese doctor on the front. Beside the picture was an article that read, "World Renowned MD Recommends Alkaline Water For Healthy Life."

Another article read, "Prominent gastroenterologist Dr. Hiromi Shinya recommends Kangen Water®."

"Here," he said, "you can have this. Take it home and read it."

He then turned on the tap and pressed a button on the machine that was sitting beside the sink.

The machine started talking. I was amazed.

"Kangen Water, 8.5."

"What's that?" I asked.

"It's the water ionizer made by Enagic®. They are the leading manufacturer of high-quality water ionizers like this one."

He pointed at the machine. "This is the Kangen Water® ionizer. It makes the healthiest water there is."

"Can I try some?" I asked.

"Sure." He gave me a cup of the water.

I was impressed. The water tasted pure and delicious.

"Very nice," I said. "The lady at the Apple Store told me that I could try this water out free for one month. How does this work?"

"Here." He handed me a big water jug. "Customers purchase a four-litre jug and can come by my store every day, and I will fill it up for free so they can drink it at home. Try this for a month and then let me know how you feel."

I was curious but needed more information. "What exactly is this water, and how is it good for you?"

He held up a picture that he pulled out of his yellow folder. "Kangen Water® detoxifies and flushes the acidic wastes out of our cells. Many people think that bottled water is good for them, but it's not. The chemicals from the plastic bottle leach into the water inside bottled water. This can't compare to Kangen Water®."

I nodded, remembering learning about the dangers of bottled water in a chemistry course. It had been surprising to learn that researchers had discovered bottled water is not free of contaminants and often has levels that exceed the allowable limits.

He continued, "Kangen Water® is also full of anti-aging antioxidants that will stop your cells from being damaged by the oxidation that leads to cancer and other diseases."

He stopped and pulled out some more papers from his folder. "Here," he said, handing me a piece of paper. "This is a testimonial from Dr. Hiromi Shinya."

It read, "I have a Kangen Water® machine in my New York medical office, and this is the water I drink and give to my patients."

He filled up the jug and then handed it to me. "Just remember, you may experience cleansing symptoms such as headaches, skin problems, and maybe temporary bowel changes. These are all normal and mean that the water is doing what it's supposed to do. You may also experience some fatigue."

I pulled the jug toward me. "Fatigue wouldn't be a problem for me."

"Why not?" he questioned.

I told him about my motorcycle accident and my brain injury and the problems I had experienced with sleep and memory since that time.

"Please keep in mind," he said. "People with a brain injury have more sensitive brains and may need to drink less of the water and build up slower." He gave me some more reading material.

Once at home I excitedly downed several glasses of Kangen Water® and sat wondering when I would start to feel tired.

I read over the reading material he had given me and learned that there were many other benefits of Kangen Water®; it can also help with diabetes, migraines, joint pain, and sleep problems.

I finally fell asleep by 10:30 p.m. but was up at 1:30 a.m.

When I awoke and saw the time, I was greatly disappointed.

This water must be a scam, I thought.

I got up and prepared myself for another difficult day. But something did feel different.

Despite only getting three hours of sleep, I had so much more energy. I couldn't believe it. I didn't feel sick. I didn't have a headache, and I didn't feel dizzy. The best feeling was that I didn't feel tired. I had never felt this with the other treatments I had tried. It was as if my batteries had been super-recharged.

I even had enough energy to work out that morning. Usually, after getting only three hours of sleep I would wake up with an extreme headache, sick and very dizzy, and be extremely tired, with no interest in working out. This was not the case that morning; I felt unusually energetic.

Once at school I continued to have a great deal of energy. The fatigue that I usually experienced during the workday did not show itself. It was like I was playing a game of hide-and-seek with fatigue. It was a good opponent and would usually find me and eventually wear me down.

But now I was winning the game and continued to hide from my adversary.

I was able to continue hiding from it for the entire day, even during my drive home. That was especially amazing for me, since I didn't even have to stop my car to clear my head. This was a first. Every day before this, I always had to stop during the drive home. Getting out and walking around a bit helped me to clear my head and feel awake enough to drive home.

The game of hide-and-seek continued at home, with me still emerging as the winner.

I wanted this feeling to continue, so I drank some more Kangen Water® as soon as I got home and then immediately got ready to go to the gym again.

Usually when I returned home, I would collapse on the couch, sick to my stomach with a splitting headache. Trying to sleep was futile, as it would rarely happen. If I were lucky enough to get some sleep, I would pay for this with a sleepless night.

A few minutes later Jen came home.

"Let's go to the gym," I said.

"Are you serious?" she said, puzzled.

I was standing smiling in the front hall. My happiness couldn't be contained.

"Absolutely."

"I figured you wouldn't want to do anything, since you didn't get much sleep last night."

I quirked an eyebrow at her. "Crazy, eh? I don't know what's happened, but there's been a change. I have so much energy today, it's unbelievable."

Jen was so pleased to see this change in me that it wasn't hard to convince her to go to the gym with me.

After the gym, I even had enough energy to go pick up a Christmas gift in the evening. But this wasn't my idea :)

By the time we got home, I was still feeling okay and had not been hit with the overwhelming feeling of fatigue I was so used to.

But as we relaxed on the couch in front of the TV, the big bang went off in my head and the fatigue set in. It was quite ironic, as Jen and I were watching our favourite TV show, *The Big Bang Theory*.

That night I was asleep by nine thirty, and for the remainder of the night I slept undisturbed until 3:30 a.m. When I awoke I was stunned. I felt very refreshed and could easily remember the vivid dreams I had that night. I felt so much better and again had so much more energy than I was used to. Lucky for me, the cleansing symptoms Jeff had warned me about only appeared as some slight headaches.

On my way home after school I stopped by the health food store. Jeff was behind the counter when I walked in.

"Hi, Jeff," I said, full of energy and life. There was no way I would forget to stop by here and get some more Kangen Water®.

"Hey, Anthony," said Jeff, smiling. "I'm glad you dropped by. I have an audio CD here for you."

"What's on it?" I asked, guessing that it had something to do with Kangen Water®.

"It's got some good information about Kangen Water®," said Jeff, handing me the CD.

I thanked him and handed him my water jugs. I was very impressed with the great service that Jeff was providing. Being able to try out this water for free and receive the help, support, and education that he was providing was very rare.

It was as if the universal energy was making it very easy for me to find another path away from my troubles. And I didn't need to depend on a doctor. This felt right, and I wanted to experience this some more.

I thanked him for his support and left the store with two large bottles of Kangen Water®, enough for one or two days, but sure I'd be back for more.

That night I got another six-hour sleep filled with many dreams. My sleep was becoming more restorative, and it was improving my energy and my mood, as well as my memory.

Things were getting so much better for me, just the way that I had hoped.

Once up, Jen and I went for our morning workout. It was so much easier to work out when I had gotten a better sleep.

I got on the stationary bike while Jen got on the treadmill right beside me.

"I know they're expensive, but I think we should seriously think about buying one of those Kangen Water® Ionizer Machines."

Jen nodded. "Well this Kangen Water® really seems to be helping your sleep, so it's probably a good idea. How about we wait and continue trying it out for the next month and then we can talk about it."

"Okay." I sighed. "It's just a lot more work having to go to this health food store every other day for more water."

"I know," agreed Jen, "Just think of it as an investment in yourself."

I agreed and then went on to finish the workout.

Seeing the improvement in my sleep and the resulting improvement in my mood quickly got Jen interested in drinking Kangen Water® as well.

Unfortunately, for me this meant stopping by the health food store had to become part of my daily routine for the next month. After only

drinking it for three weeks, we agreed to purchase a Kangen Water®
machine.

As I continued to drink Kangen Water®, I usually got about six hours
of sleep each night.

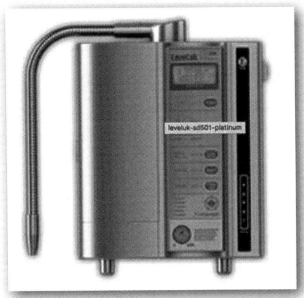

The Leveluk SD501 to make Kangen Water®

SCIENCE NOTES

The following information came from several sources, as outlined in the
references at the end of this book.

Kangen Water® is a delicious, healing alkaline water made by
Enagic®, one of the leading manufacturers of high-quality water ionizers in Japan.

Kangen Water® assists the body in creating the necessary balance or
homeostasis in order to help the body heal itself.

One of the alkaline water machines that is made by Enagic® and produces Kangen Water® is called the Leveluk SD501.

The Enagic® Leveluk SD501 is considered the "Gold Standard" in all water ionizers.

The water produced is full of anti-aging antioxidants, is very hydrating, and detoxifies, flushing toxins and acidic wastes out of the cells. One's health is greatly improved when the toxins and acidic wastes are removed from the body.

This machine removes many harmful chemicals from tap water and produces a healthier water through the process of electrolysis.

The electrolysis process separates ordinary tap water (H_2O) into two separate streams. Half of the separated water becomes acidic with an abundance of (H^+) molecules, while the other becomes alkaline with an abundance of (OH^-) molecules. The alkaline (OH^-) Kangen Water® is used for drinking purposes.

The Kangen Water® machine will enable someone to make healthy alkaline drinking water right in their home that is antioxidant, mineral-rich, pure, and safe. This water contains important minerals such as calcium, magnesium, potassium, and sodium. The Enagic® Kangen Water® ionizer machine will keep these minerals intact, unlike many other water filtration systems that filter out these helpful minerals.

As we age and experience more of the health challenges that come with life, the goal for many is to feel better and find ways to improve their health.

Many people feel the struggle of maintaining an optimum level of health, despite the fact that they try to eat healthy, exercise regularly, and take various health supplements. It is our lifestyle choices that have the greatest impact on our health.

Many health problems we experience are caused by mild acidosis. This is a condition when your body fluids contain too much acid.

Acidosis occurs when your kidneys and lungs can't keep your body's pH in balance. Kangen Water® can improve this condition.

When your body is too acidic, it will start taking important minerals from your bones and vital organs to neutralize the acid, which is then eliminated from the body. The loss of important body minerals such as calcium, magnesium, potassium, and sodium can go on for some time until it reaches unhealthy levels, causing acidosis.

PH Scale of Common Substances

Most Acidic -	0 -	Battery Acid
	1	
	2 -	Lemon Juice
	3 -	Vinegar
	4 -	Tomato Juice
	5 -	Black Coffee
	6 -	Milk
Neutral	7 -	Water
	8 -	Seawater
	9 -	Baking Soda
	10 -	Milk of magnesia
	11 -	Ammonia
	12 -	Soapy water
	13 -	Lye
Most Alkaline	14	

The body naturally flushes out and removes acids and toxins through sweating, urination, and defecation. However, the body can become overwhelmed when there is too much acid and toxicity. Fat cells are then produced to serve as toxic waste storage cells. As a final line of defence, the fat cells help maintain life by storing toxins and excess acid.

There are a variety of health problems caused by acidosis, including fatigue, sleep problems, low energy, headaches, migraines, confusion, poor concentration, emotional problems, obesity, diabetes, asthma, arthritis, muscular aches, neck pain, back pain, knee pain, joint problems, eczema, psoriasis, acid reflux, high blood pressure, and high cholesterol. In order to improve your alkalinity and overcome acidosis, you should drink plenty of Kangen Water®, regularly check your pH, and avoid acidic foods and drinks as much as possible.

Drinking Kangen Water® will fight acidosis by helping your body flush out toxins and acid from your body.

It will slow the aging process and increase the absorption of vitamins and minerals as well as oxygenate your blood.

Drinking Kangen Water® also helps to increase the amount of water that gets into the cells. The water inside the Kangen Water® Ionizer undergoes a change that reduces the size of the water molecular cluster by two-thirds. Smaller water clusters are more able to penetrate the cellular membranes, enhancing tissue repair and waste removal.

The pH of the body is balanced by drinking Kangen Water® on a regular basis. The pH scale ranges from 0 to 14. It measures how acidic or basic (alkaline) a substance is. A pH of 7 is neutral. A pH less than 7 is acidic. A pH greater than 7 is basic or alkaline.

Kangen Water® raises the pH of your drinking water. It does this by ionizing or splitting the water molecule (H_2O) resulting in the ions' H^+ (hydrogen with a positive electrical charge), and OH^- (hydroxyl ion with a negative electrical charge), as well as ionic alkaline minerals. This abundance of OH^- ions increases the bicarbonate buffers in the blood, balancing the pH of the body and neutralizing and excreting acids and toxins.

The abundance of hydroxyl ions ($OH-$) in strong, fresh Kangen Water® have free electrons which are readily donated to unstable oxygen free radicals, resulting in stable oxygen molecules. Drinking Kangen

Water® on a regular basis will increase the amount of dissolved oxygen in the blood. More oxygen in the blood provides us with mental alertness and gives us more energy to cope with the daily challenges.

Please visit my website at https://anthonyaquan-assee.com for more information on Kangen Water®.

Rethink, Redo, Rewire

HUMANS ENGAGE IN HABITUAL BEHAVIOURS and routines. In other words, we usually like to do the same thing on a consistent basis. We eat the same foods, drink the same drinks, take the same route to work, or deal with our daily problems in a similar way. It helps us to feel more comfortable as we go through our life on autopilot. We have dozens of habits that often help us move forward during our day. Some of these habits also involve our health care. This might appear in our lives as having the same health-care providers, choosing to have the same medical treatments, and taking the same medications at the same time and often in the same place.

People who have overcome a major health crisis have been able to rethink, redo, and rewire themselves for success. What did they do that was different?

First, they didn't lose hope and accept the finality of their diagnosis. They changed their thoughts and beliefs, which resulted in new behaviours, attitudes, and habits. In addition, they didn't accept the most likely outcome as outlined by their doctors. They did not see themselves as victims of their condition, because they knew they were part of the solution. Their belief and hope were two sides of the same coin.

Trying alternative treatments was a change to my habitual way of turning to conventional medicine for help. This involved changing my thoughts and beliefs about alternative treatments. This was not that hard to do, since I had basically given up on conventional medicine with the same treatments, the same medications, and the same poor results. I was ready for a change. This made it easier for me to accept the possibilities of alternative treatments, and a clear intention was born.

The energy of this heightened awareness was greater than what was hardwired into my brain. With this change, my body became ready to accept the healing triggered by different alternative treatments. Hence, I rewired myself.

The greatest force in the human body is the natural drive of the body to heal itself, and it is your thinking that drives this force.

Health is not something that you need to acquire; it is something you already have. Don't let your thoughts and beliefs interfere with it.

Everything begins with a belief. "As you think, so shall you be" (Dr. W. Dyer). Your thoughts and beliefs are the energy that direct your journey in life.

EPILOGUE

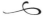

THE WIDE VARIETY OF ALTERNATIVE treatments that are available can be seen as a menu of possibilities for improving one's health.

Exploring different treatment options addresses the different needs that we all have. An alternative treatment is generally used instead of conventional medical treatments. However, they can also be used alongside other alternative treatments or in conjunction with various medical treatments. This multimodal approach can enable the treatments to build on one another's possibilities. It is important to note that different needs require different tools.

Always be sure to discuss with your doctor any treatments that you are thinking of using.

I have learned in my recovery the importance of working alongside a team of healing professionals to serve as a guide in one's recovery.

Work with your health-care professionals to help you make informed decisions about the best treatments for you. A commitment to the healing process is very important.

Throughout the process of healing myself, I learned that I am responsible for acting and taking care of myself. I have learned to empower myself so that I can direct my own healing and be an advocate in my healing journey.

In the years following my motorcycle accident, I had to use so many different medications to deal with many health problems. These included sleep problems, anxiety, and depression, as well as problems with the rest of my body. All of these drugs came with many different side effects. The medications made me feel better temporarily, but in time the same symptoms and problems came back. This was because the medications were not addressing the root of my problems.

No longer do I need to take any medication. Basically, the most difficult problems (sleep, anxiety, depression) I experienced after sustaining my brain injuries no longer require me to get help from conventional medicine. I learned that there wasn't a "cure-all" for my problems. Instead, I learned to manage quite well using alternative treatments.

Being drug-free enables my body to focus on healing instead of expending the effort needed to detoxify and remove drugs and other chemicals.

I am inspired by people who are able to start over and build themselves up and focus on being a person of value, those who don't need an audience to know they have value, and those who aren't scared to walk on the road less travelled.

In this world you will encounter many problems and challenges, with many lessons to be learned. To realize your full potential, surround yourself with those who support your decisions and do not discourage you from pursing potential avenues toward healing. Recovering your capacity to function more effectively after a health crisis requires the support and love of those close to you. It is through our interactions with others that we discover ourselves.

Looking back, it seems as if my personal experiences were carefully planned to prepare me for what lay ahead. It was as if I had an invisible team of strategic planners working on my behalf, without my knowledge, to ensure the correct sequence of my life's events. In order to grow and continue to move forward, I had to Rethink, Redo, and Rewire my brain.

"He who conquers himself is the mightiest warrior."

—Confucius (551–479 B.C.E.)

Anthony Aquan-Assee, MEd, graduated from the University of Toronto with a bachelor of science and four years later received a bachelor of education from Nipissing University in North Bay, Ontario. In 1997, Anthony was in a motorcycle accident and slipped into a coma for two weeks. In the year 2000, he received the prestigious Courage to Come Back Award from the Centre for Addictions and Mental Health in Toronto.

Anthony went on to graduate from the University of Toronto with a Master of Education. He is the author of *Second Life, Second Chance: A Teacher's Chronicle of Despair, Recovery, and Triumph*, *Starting Over: A Survivor's Guide*, and a fantasy novel titled *Vendeka's Creed*. In 2009, Anthony won an Eric Hoffer Award for Independent Publishing. His writing is influenced by "seeing the light" after a near-death experience. He works in Toronto, Canada, as a teacher, author, and motivational speaker.

REFERENCES

⤚

N. Doidge. *The Brain That Changes Itself*. New York: Penguin Books, 2007.

N. Doidge. *The Brain's Way of Healing*. New York: Penguin Books, 2016.

W. Dyer. *There's a Spiritual Solution to Every Problem*. New York: HarperCollins Publishers 2001.

J. Dispenza. *You Are the Placebo*. New York: Hay House, Inc., 2014.

GENERAL WEBSITES
M. Smith, L. Robinson, and R. Segal. "How much sleep do we really need?" (2017)
Retrieved from https://www.helpguide.org/home-pages/sleep.htm

G. Johnson. (2010) Sleep Disorders.
Retrieved from http://www.tbiguide.com/sleepdisorders.html

Sleep Disorders (2017) Retrieved from https://sleepfoundation.org/sleep-disorders-problems

Mental Fatigue (2014) Retrieved from http://www.betterhealthusa.com/public/235.cfm

C. Armstrong, "Emotional changes following brain injury: psychological and neurological components of depression, denial and anxiety," *Journal of Rehabilitation*, April-June, 1991.

M. Smith, L. Robinson, R. Segal. (2017) Sleep Disorders and Problems. Retrieved from https://www.helpguide.org/articles/sleep/sleep-disorders-and-sleeping-problems.htm?pdf=true

NEUROFEEDBACK
K. Shue. (2015) Neurofeedback. Retrieved from: http://www.brainandhealth.com/neurofeedback

How Does Neuroptimal Work? (2016). Retrieved from https://neuroptimal.com/learn/178-2/

What is Neurofeedback (2017). Retrieved from http://www.eeginfo.com/what-is-neurofeedback.jsp

CRANIAL ELECTROTHERAPY STIMULATION (CES)
D. Kirsch. (2008). CES For Mild Traumatic Brain Injury. Practical PAIN MANAGEMENT
Retrieved from http://www.stress.org/wp-content/uploads/CES_Research/kirsch_brain_injury.pdf

Daniel L. Kirsch, Jeff A. Marksberry, Larry R. Price, Francine H. Nichols, Katherine T. Platoni. (2015). Cranial Electrotherapy

Stimulation: Treatment of Pain and Headache in Military Population. Retrieved From: https://www.practicalpainmanagement.com/treatments/interventional/stimulators/cranial-electrotherapy-stimulation-treatment-pain-headache

What is Cranial Electrotherapy Stimulation? (2016). **Retrieved from** http://www.drmueller-healthpsychology.com/what_is_ces.html

LASER THERAPY
Meditech International Incorporated (2013). Bio Flex Laser Therapy.The safe and effective way to eliminate pain. (Brochure). Ontario, Canada. Author.

We Are Made of Light: Scientific Evidence. (2014)
Retrieved from http://humansarefree.com/2014/04/we-are-made-of-light-scientific-evidence.html

M. Eisner. Laser Therapy. (2015).
Retrieved from http://www.integratedmedicine.ca/team_member/laser-therapy-2/

Benjamin Yuen, Fred Kahn. Laser Therapy for Concussion. (2013).
Retrieved from http://www.canadianchiropractor.ca/techniques/laser-therapy-for-concussion-2561

KANGEN WATER®
Who is Enagic® USA (2016). Retrieved from https://www.enagic.com/enagic.php

What is Kangen Water® from Enagic®? (2011). Retrieved from https://www.enagic.com/blog/what-is-kangen-water-from-enagic/

What is Kangen Water®? Retrieved from BestWaterHealing.com

Why Can't You Lose Weight? (2000).
Retrieved from   http://www.vitalearthminerals.com/category-s/1907.htm

S. E. Gould (2012). What makes things acid: The pH scale. Scientific American.
Retrieved From:
https://blogs.scientificamerican.com/lab-rat/what-makes-things-acid-the-ph-scale/

70410717R10061

Made in the USA
Columbia, SC
06 May 2017